Shelly Schonho

home • Caregiver • *guide*

UPDATED
EDITION

SIMON & KOLZ PUBLISHING
DUBUQUE, IOWA

Always consult and follow the advice of a licensed health care practitioner and comply with the law applicable in your jurisdiction. This publication is intended to serve as a general statement of information currently available; however, it is not a substitute for the diagnosis, advice or guidance of a physician, psychiatrist or other health care practitioner. Each patient's condition and circumstances are unique. A publication cannot be individualized, address every medical need, practice or therapy, assure compliance with all laws, answer questions or correct misunderstandings. Alternative practices may be required under the circumstances, or information may become outdated as laws and medical opinions and practices change rapidly. The publisher is not engaged in the practice of law, medicine or any related field and is not responsible for the completeness or accuracy of the information presented or referred to by the author. It is the responsibility of an attending health care practitioner to decide what care is appropriate under specific circumstances, and as always it is the responsibility of the care provider to comply with all applicable laws.

Illustrations: Paula Schulting
Cover and interior design and layout: Imagine Design Studio, Kelly Fassbinder

ISBN: 1-58254-035-7

Printed in the United States of America

Introduction

Being a Caregiver

You have found yourself in a very challenging position. You have either voluntarily chosen to care for another person, are anticipating the need, or are obligated in some way to perform care in the home. The majority of people prefer to be in their own home setting where their surroundings are familiar, their privacy is respected, and they can maintain some control over their lives. Being at home also allows people to keep in closer contact with extended family members, their churches, and community organizations.

We will prepare you to meet the challenge by teaching you how to become a skilled and sensitive caregiver.

Our goal throughout this book is to provide you with simple explanations and instructions so that you are not overwhelmed with medical terminology and complicated procedures. You will also be given practical guidance on learning to recognize your own needs and the importance of sharing problems with others.

This guide provides information on how to utilize available support services, such as home health aides, housekeeping companions, and adult day care centers. By utilizing part-time and alternate caregivers, the patient can remain engaged in life and you will be able to relax and enjoy your own personal interests outside of care giving. The knowledge you obtain from this book will promote the maximum independence not only for the patient, but also for yourself and any family involved.

You will learn through this experience that the wholeness of the human body is not only physical health, but also mental, spiritual, and social well- being. The best teachers will be those you are caring for. It is through them that you will find great rewards and an understanding of the human spirit.

By providing assistance to those in need, you are taking on an important task. The number of people being cared for in the home is on the rise, so know that you are not alone. This book is an offering to you. It is presented with the wisdom and experience of many health care providers, both medical and non-medical.

Armed with the basic knowledge and understanding of providing care in the home, both you and your patient will benefit tremendously. A sure path to the healing process is found in the security and comforts of one's own home and with the love and compassion of a caregiver. We truly do understand your needs and feel fortunate to be able to share this information with you. We hope in some way this book will make your life just a little bit easier.

A note about the use of terms and pronouns in this guide: We will refer to the person you are taking care of as the patient throughout. We will refer to you as the caregiver.

In order to avoid awkward uses of pronouns throughout (i.e., he/she each time we speak of the patient), we will use the masculine "he" in odd-numbered chapters; the feminine "she" in even-numbered chapters. Of course, where there is a need for a specific gender, we will use the appropriate pronoun.

Chapter 1
Safety

Feeling safe and secure is not an entitlement; it is a necessity—especially in our home. Your patient depends on you to provide an environment that is free of danger. In this chapter you will find some basic safety instructions that will give you the confidence of knowing that you have made the home as safe as possible.

Patients cared for in the home should always be under the supervision of a doctor. Have a clear idea of what you must do medically. Ask the doctor for written condition-specific instructions and a list of all medications. Emergency phone numbers should be in large print and posted next to the telephone so if the need arises, you can obtain help quickly.

Personal Hygiene

No matter the condition or the age of the patient, certain practices should be so routine that you do not even have to think about doing them.

- Hand washing: Always wash your hands with soap under running water before and after you touch the patient. Work up a good lather and rub your hands together vigorously for a full minute. Rinse your hands and the bar of soap well after each use. Dry your hands with a clean cloth or paper towel. Assist your patient in washing his hands before eating and after toileting. If it is too difficult for the patient to get to a sink, a plastic bowl with warm soapy water and a pitcher of rinse water will work. Wear disposable gloves when helping with toileting or changing a wound bandage. Disposable gloves can be purchased at most pharmacies or medical supply stores.

- Hand sanitizers: This is a liquid that destroys germs on your hands. No soap, water, or towels are needed. Hand sanitizers can be purchased at most variety stores, and include brand names such as Dial and Purell.

Infection Control and Waste Disposal

When sickness occurs, it is much easier to get an infection because the body cannot fight off germs if it is in a weakened condition.

- Have a box of tissues within easy reach for the patient's nose and throat discharges.
- Immediately dispose of all soiled bandages and used tissues in a plastic-lined wastebasket which you can close up without touching the contents.
- Urine, stool, vomit, and blood should be flushed down the toilet.
- Change soiled linens and bedclothes promptly. They may be washed and dried in the usual manner unless you have been instructed otherwise.
- Clean up spills immediately.
- Wash all fresh fruits and vegetables thoroughly before serving. All meat should be cooked thoroughly.

☞ *Remember:*

GOOD HAND WASHING IS THE NUMBER ONE WEAPON IN STOPPING THE SPREAD OF DISEASE.

Preparing the Environment/ Accident Prevention

Often it is necessary to rearrange a room in the house in order to meet the safety needs of the patient. The ideal room is pleasant, well lit, uncluttered, quiet, and well-ventilated. A ground floor room is preferred—assuming there is access to a bathroom—as the location eases the workload of the caregiver and also allows the patient to be near household activity. Provide a bedside table to hold a glass of water, some tissues, and other personal items.

- Keep the furnishings simple but do not remove familiar objects that soften the room or are pleasing to the patient.
- Bedpan and urinal should be in easy reach.
- Never clutter the bedside with unnecessary items as this increases the risk of accidents.
- A night-light in the room will provide a sense of security and many times can help the patient avoid confusion or disorientation.
- A bell or whistle should be within easy reach of the patient to be used to call for help.
- A phone or medical alert device should be available if the patient is ever left unattended in the home. The medical alert device is an emergency calling system that is worn as a necklace or carried in the pocket. Ask the doctor for details.
- A carbon monoxide detector installed in the home can detect and alert inhabitants to the presence of this highly poisonous, odorless gas.
- During times of severe weather, decide in advance a safe area of the home where you will go with the patient. Be prepared by having working flashlights, blankets, drinking water, and snacks available in the selected area. The plan should be shared with all caregivers.

- The patient should wear non-slip footwear whenever he is standing or walking.
- Caution: Pets underfoot can easily cause falls.

Living Room

1. Furniture: Couches and chairs that have arms and are not too low are the easiest to sit in.
2. Lighting: Always have additional lighting where reading or special procedures will take place.
3. Passageways: All hallways and doorways should be clear and free of excess furniture, electrical cords, and other unnecessary objects.
4. Rugs: Remove throw rugs as these are easily tripped over.

Stairways

1. Handrails: Handrails should be added to all stairways for support. They can be purchased at most home improvement stores. A professional should install these to insure that they are attached securely to the wall.
2. Flooring: Add a bright colored strip to the first and last step as this is where most tripping occurs. Repair or replace any flooring in poor condition.
3. Lighting: Add additional lighting if necessary so that steps can be seen easily.
4. Shoes: The patient should wear supportive shoes when walking up stairs. Open backed slippers cause many falls.

Bathroom

1. Rugs: Remove all throw rugs.
2. Bars: Add grab bars near the toilet and bathtub. These can be purchased at home improvement, hardware, and medical supply stores.

3 Benches: A bath bench or chair and hand-held shower are excellent aids in making bath time easier. They can be purchased at hardware and medical supply stores.
4 Mats: The bottom of the tub should have a bath mat or nonslip strips to avoid slipping.

Bedroom

1 Night-light: A night-light is essential in every bedroom to prevent disorientation when getting up during the night.
2 Bed: Consider the purchase or rental of a hospital-style bed with side rails to prevent accidental falls out of bed. Side rails can give the patient a sense of security as well as ease the mind of the caregiver. Check with the patient's doctor about Medicare coverage for this expense.
3 Chair: Provide a firm chair with arms to make sitting and dressing easier.
4 Lighting: Add additional lighting near the patient's bed where reading or special procedures will take place.
5 Storage: Organize all supplies to avoid clutter.
6 Telephone: A telephone should be at the patient's bedside. Instruct the patient and all caregivers on the use of 911 for emergencies.
7 Toilet: Consider getting a portable toilet (commode) to place next to the bed.
8 Rugs: Use rubber pads, carpet tape, or tacks to keep all area rugs in place. Remove all throw rugs.

Remember:

SECURITY IN ONE'S SURROUNDING REDUCES UNNECESSARY STRESS AND ANXIETY.

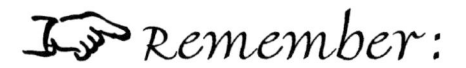

Fire Safety

Fires in the home can often be prevented if some basic safety measures are followed. Often we do not foresee this tragedy as something that can happen to us. However, because the patient's vision, hearing, mobility, and ability to make decisions are often impaired, the following steps are important:

- The entire household should have a plan to get out of the house in case of fire. Pathways should be clear. Every room must have at least one unblocked doorway.
- Do not smoke in bed or with oxygen usage. Many fires are started this way.
- Space heaters can be very dangerous. Keep them at least three feet away from people and objects. Never dry clothes on space heaters.
- Install a smoke detector on every level of the home. Test all detectors once a month.
- Repair or throw out frayed or damaged electrical cords. Unplug appliances when they are not in use. Never place an electrical appliance near a sink, tub, or shower area.
- Removing soot and dust from the heating system will help prevent chimney and flue fires.
- Avoid the use of extension cords when possible. If needed, use a heavy one.
- Supervise the use of the range and other appliances that may cause injury or accident.

☞ Remember:

SMOKE DETECTORS CAN ALERT YOU EVEN BEFORE FIRE IS PRESENT.

Decreased Sensation and Burns

Along with age, illness, or disease—such as diabetes or circulatory problems—the sensation of touch often decreases. A person with shakiness, weakness, or poor muscle control has difficulty holding a cup steady. A frequent cause of burns is the spilling of hot liquids onto the skin.

- Swallowing coffee or soup that is too hot can cause serious injury to the mouth and throat. Let very hot liquids cool for a few minutes before you give them to the patient.
- You as the caregiver should test the bath water for temperature safety before assisting the patient to enter the bath.
- Heating pads should be used with caution on the lower settings only and checked frequently. The patient should not use a heating pad longer than twenty minutes at a time.
- Steam vaporizers can help make breathing easier, but the vapor is hot enough to cause burns, and if tipped onto the patient can cause serious injury. Put the vaporizer on a sturdy table, far enough away from the patient's bed or chair to prevent accidentally bumping into it.

Remember:

FOOD SHOULD BE SERVED WARM, NOT HOT.

Oxygen Usage

Special equipment may be required in the home for patient care. Oxygen is frequently ordered by the doctor. It is managed and supplied by a company or hospital that is trained in the use of oxygen equipment. The supplier is responsible for setting everything up in the home and will give you detailed instructions specific to the patient's needs. The doctor's office or a home health care nurse will arrange this. Since oxygen is considered a medication, instructions should be followed exactly as ordered. These tips will help to ensure the safe use of oxygen:

1 Do not smoke or allow others to smoke in the home, as oxygen is a gas and can explode if it is near a flame or spark.
2 "No Smoking" signs should be placed outside the patient's bedroom door, and on the outside of the main entrance into the home. The oxygen supplier will provide these signs.
3 Oxygen tubing should trail behind the patient when he is walking to prevent tripping over it.
4 Avoid using electrical equipment, such as hair dryers or razors, when oxygen is in use.

in**sight**

Trust your instinct if you find yourself in a situation that requires a quick decision.

Summary

In summary, safety is an essential requirement when caring for a patient. There are supplies available to make the home a safe environment. Many accidents can be prevented with a little forethought.

Chapter 2
Personal Hygiene

Hygiene cares such as bathing, dressing, and care of the hair, nails, mouth and skin will be a part of the patient's daily routine. How often the patient bathes and changes clothes will depend on her needs, wishes, and cultural beliefs. By being respectful and considerate of her feelings, you will establish a trust that can make this time a positive experience.

Cleanliness plays an important role in the way a patient feels about herself. A clean body will provide a feeling of confidence and improved self-image. The patient should be encouraged to help with her personal care as much as she is able, even if it is just washing her own hands and face. This will promote independence and feelings of accomplishment.

If the patient is unable to assist, it will be up to you to provide the needed care or make arrangements for alternate care. Home health care agencies provide services to the chronically ill, disabled, or recuperating patient in the home. These agencies offer assistance from a variety of health care professionals. See page 116 for a listing of Home Health Services.

Home health aides provide a wonderful service for both the patient and the caregiver. The patient is usually very accepting of this service because there is little disruption in her lifestyle and it provides her with additional social interaction.

Having a home health aide in the home will allow you, the caregiver, to be alleviated of some of the patient's hygiene responsibilities as well as provide you with some time for yourself. Home health aides can help the patient with:

- Bathing
- Dressing
- Nail care
- Light housekeeping
- Exercise assistance
- Toileting

This chapter will give you the information needed to perform personal care. Keep in mind that bath time provides you with an excellent opportunity to look at the patient's body. Often the caregiver is the first to notice a change in the skin, or a sudden difference in the way the patient is able to move her arms and legs.

At first you may feel a little uncomfortable giving a bath, brushing teeth, or trimming toenails. This is a very natural way to feel. The patient may be embarrassed, as grooming was once a very personal task performed in the privacy of her own bathroom. A good story, funny joke or a favorite song will help to relax and lessen some of the anxiety you both may be feeling.

Bathing

Bathing cleans the skin, is very relaxing, provides exercise for bones and joints, and improves circulation. Baths should be quick, but thorough. Long baths can be very tiring, as well as drying to the skin. There are three basic types of baths:

1 The bed bath is ideal for someone who is too ill, weak, or physically unable to leave the bed. The entire bath is done with the patient lying in bed.
2 For the patient who is physically capable of getting into and out of the tub alone, or with little assistance, a tub bath or shower is appropriate. Grab bars should be installed first.

3 A partial bath can be offered to any patient. It can be done in bed, or at the bathroom sink. A partial bath includes washing the face, hands, armpits, genital area, buttocks, and the back. You may prefer to do a partial bath on days when a complete bath is not given.

☞ Remember:

ENCOURAGE THE PATIENT TO PARTICIPATE WITH HER PERSONAL CARE AS MUCH AS SHE IS ABLE.

Before you start:

1 Close all windows to avoid drafts.
2 Pull the shades down or close the curtains to provide privacy.
3 Assist the patient to the bathroom or offer the urinal or bed pan, as warm water often stimulates the need to urinate.
4 Look around. Are there any hazards that could interfere with the safety of the patient during the bath? If there are, remove them.
5 Make sure the room and water temperature are comfortable.
6 Tell the patient what you will be doing. Collect the items you will need, and wash your hands thoroughly.
7 Be alert to any unusual conditions of the skin, such as redness, swelling, sores, rashes, and unusual bruising. Report noticed skin changes to the doctor. Refer to Chapter 7, Comfort Measures, for more information on skin care.

Bed Bath

What you will need:

1 Large plastic bowl or container one-half full of warm water
2 Liquid or bar soap. Soaps containing deodorants and perfumes may cause unnecessary dryness or skin irritation.

3 Two washcloths, two towels
4 One lightweight blanket or beach towel
5 Clean change of clothing
6 Lotion
7 Deodorant

Put all items on a nearby end table or night stand before beginning.

Remember these simple rules:

1 Lower the bed rail (if this applies), but do not leave the bedside while the railing is down.
2 Protect the bedding with towels or waterproof pads. These can be purchased at most variety stores. A towel folded lengthwise, placed under the arms and legs, will provide additional protection to the bedding.
3 Start at the head and work down.
4 Uncover and wash small areas at a time.
5 When drying, pat the skin. Do not rub.

Eyes: Use plain water. Do not use soap. Wipe the closed eye from the side closest to the nose, moving outward. Use a different part of the washcloth for the other eye.

Face and Ears: You may or may not use soap. If the skin is very dry, use plain water. Rinse and dry well.

After you wash the eyes, face, and ears, remove the patient's gown or clothing. Cover her with the blanket or beach towel.

Remember:

EXPOSE ONLY THE AREA OF THE BODY YOU ARE WASHING. KEEP THE REST WELL COVERED.

Neck, Chest and Abdomen: Wash, rinse, and dry well. Pay special attention to skin folds and creases. Skin breakdown can occur in areas that remain moist.

Arms and Hands: Using long, firm strokes, wash the arms and armpits. Rinse and dry well. Have the patient put her hand into the warm, soapy water and wiggle her fingers for a minute or two. This is comforting and cleans the fingers and hands well.

Legs and Feet: Have the patient bend her leg at the knee if she is able. It will make washing easier. Using long strokes, wash and rinse well. Place the foot in the warm soapy water for a minute or two. Wash the foot and between the toes with the washcloth. Rinse. Gently slide a dry towel back and forth between each toe to dry.

Back and Buttocks: Help the patient roll onto her side. Adjust the bath blanket to expose the back and buttocks. Wash the back using long firm strokes. Rinse and dry. With one hand lift up the upper buttocks. With the other hand, wash the anal area front to back using a single stroke. Using a different part of the washcloth, repeat until clean. Avoid the genital area at this time.

Change the water and use the clean washcloth and towel now.

Genitals: This area should always be washed last. In a female, wipe the genital area from the front to the back with one stroke. Continue, using a different section of the washcloth with each stroke until clean.

In a male patient, wash the penis from the tip towards the body. Then wash the scrotum. Rinse and dry well.

After bathing, the patient may enjoy a back massage as this relaxes muscles and stimulates circulation.

1 Rub lotion between your hands to warm it.
2 Massage the back for 3 to 5 minutes, using firm, circular strokes.

There are times when a back massage could be harmful, such as in the case of injuries to the muscles and bones of the upper body. If in doubt about this, check with the patient's doctor first.

insight

The touch of your hand can reach someone's heart.

Tub Bath or Shower

A patient able to get into and out of the tub should do so very slowly. Falls can occur when the patient is rushed. A weak or disabled patient should have a shower chair to sit on. A chair can be purchased at a medical supply store. A commode chair with the pan removed will also work. Hand-held spray attachments make showering easier. A grab bar is a helpful bath aid and will give the patient a sense of security when transferring into and out of the tub or shower.

Remember these simple rules:

1 A non-skid bath mat should be placed in the tub or shower unit.
2 Have all needed items in reach of the patient.
3 Make sure the temperature of the bath water is comfortable before the patient gets in.

4 Do not use oils in the bath water, as oils will make the tub surfaces slippery.
5 Do not leave the patient unattended while she is in the bathtub or shower.
6 Drain the bath water before allowing the patient to get out of the tub.
7 Clean the tub or shower unit after each use to avoid the spread of germs.

Dressing

- Pajamas or gowns made of cotton or flannel are best for night time wear, and for the patient who spends a large part of the day in bed.
- Trousers or pants with elastic waistlines are less binding and are easier to get on and off.
- Loose fitting tops that button in the front or back are easier to put on and take off than those that pull over the head.
- Hospital-type gowns that tie in the back work best for the patient who requires total care.
- Large buttons, snaps, zippers or Velcro closures may allow the patient to dress independently. A seamstress can alter a patient's existing clothing to meet special needs. Several manufacturers make adaptive clothing that can be ordered through a catalog.*
- Soft cotton socks with some stretch are comfortable and easy to put on.
- The patient may feel chilly when you do not. A cardigan sweater or lap blanket will help her feel more comfortable.
- For a patient who is wheelchair bound, avoid loose hanging clothing that can get caught in the wheels.

*An internet site providing links to adaptive clothing sources is www.makoa.org/clothing.htm

Care of the Eyes, Ears, Mouth, Hair, Feet, and Nails

Eyes

It is important for the caregiver to have an understanding of eye care and know what to report to the doctor.

Symptoms to report:

- Pain or pressure in the eye
- Unusual redness or itchiness
- Seeing dark spots or halos
- Increased matter or drainage from the eye
- Sudden change in vision, such as blurring or double vision

If the doctor orders eye drops:

1 Wash your hands before and after administering the drops. Have a tissue handy.
2 Clean the eyelid and eyelashes with a warm washcloth if there is any drainage or matter present. *(See page 12 for cleaning the eyes.)*
3 Follow the doctor's instructions exactly as ordered.
4 The patient may lie on her back, or sit with her head tilted back slightly.
5 Hold the dropper or container one-half inch from the eyeball. Do not touch the eyeball or eyelashes with your hand or the dropper.
6 Pull down on the skin just above the cheekbone. Instruct the patient to look upward, and instill the drops at the base of the white portion of the eyeball. (If a second eye drop is needed in the same eye, wait five minutes before administering.)

Ears

Besides cleaning the ears, little additional care is needed. A small visible amount of wax is normal. Avoid putting anything into the ear canal—including cotton swabs—as this can cause a hard buildup of wax to press on the eardrum, resulting in pain and hearing loss.

☞ Remember:

CLEANSE ONLY THAT PORTION OF THE EAR THAT YOU CAN REACH WITH YOUR WASHCLOTH.

Symptoms to report:

- Visible drainage from the ear or seen on the pillow case
- Redness and pain
- Pulling at the ear
- Sudden hearing loss or a ringing sound in the ear

☞ Remember:

ALWAYS REMOVE HEARING AIDS BEFORE YOU WASH THE EARS. A SIGNIFICANT WEIGHT LOSS OR GAIN CAN CHANGE THE WAY A HEARING AID FITS AND CAN EVEN CAUSE SORES IN THE EARS. HEARING AIDS SHOULD BE CHECKED BY A PROFESSIONAL EVERY SIX MONTHS OR SOONER IF THE PATIENT IS HAVING PROBLEMS.

If the doctor orders ear drops:

1 Wash your hands before and after you put the drops into the ear.

2 Warm the medication first by holding the bottle in your hands for two minutes. Medication that is too cool can cause dizziness.
3 Have the patient lay on her side with the affected ear turned up.
4 Fill the dropper as you were instructed.
5 Hold onto the upper portion of the ear and pull upward and back. This straightens the passageway into the ear.
7 Instill the drops.
8 Wait five minutes before turning the head to the other side. This will prevent the medication from running back out.

When using ear drops, avoid getting water into the ears during bathing, showering, or shampooing. Ear plugs can be worn as an extra precaution. The doctor's office or local drug store has ear plugs available.

Mouth

It is important not to overlook the mouth when performing personal care. Poorly fitting dentures, missing or cracked teeth, cavities and mouth sores can greatly affect the patient's ability to eat, drink, and talk. Bad breath is also a common problem that can be reduced or eliminated with good oral hygiene.

If the patient has her own teeth:

1 Brush the teeth, tongue, and gums every morning and night.
2 Use a toothbrush that is soft, non-frayed, and rounded. It should be small enough to reach the back teeth.
3 The toothpaste should contain fluoride.
4 Floss the teeth daily.

Brushing the patient's teeth:

1 Assist the patient to the bathroom sink, if she is able.
2 If brushing the patient's teeth in bed, first put her into a sitting position.
3 Offer a sip of water to moisten the mouth.
4 Wet the brush and put a small amount of toothpaste onto the brush.
5 Place a small basin or bowl under the patient's chin.
6 Direct the toothbrush bristles toward the gum line. Brush the front, back, and sides of the teeth using gentle, short strokes. Brush for two full minutes.

The mouth should be rinsed thoroughly with water following brushing.

Brushing the patient's dentures:

Take special care when handling the dentures. They are easily broken if dropped and are costly to replace. Observe for dentures in need of repair as they can cause painful sores and swelling in the mouth. Keep in mind that significant weight loss or gain can lead to improperly fitting dentures.

1 Place the washcloth in the bottom of the sink to protect the dentures should they slip from your hands while cleaning them.
2 Brush the dentures as you would regular teeth. Toothpaste, denture cleansers, or tablets can be used.
3 Rinse well. Gently brush the patient's gums and tongue before replacing the dentures.
4 Each night, place the dentures in a denture cup after brushing and cover with cold water. Store them in a safe place until morning.

Flossing:

1 Use twelve inches or so of waxed or unwaxed floss.
2 Wrap it around one finger of each hand.
3 Slide the floss between the teeth down to the gum line, using a gentle back and forth motion.

Oral swabs should be used for the patient who is unable to sit up in bed, or unable to rinse her mouth out.

☞ Remember:

GOOD CARE OF THE MOUTH AND TEETH WILL PROMOTE BETTER NUTRITION, AND ENABLE THE PATIENT TO COMMUNICATE MORE EFFECTIVELY.

Hair

You should brush or comb the patient's hair daily. It improves appearance, stimulates the scalp, and brings dirt and oils onto the hair strands where they can be washed away. The hair, including beards, should be shampooed as often as needed or preferred by the patient. Select a shampoo that best fits the patient's hair type. Use a conditioner if the hair tangles easily, is long, or very dry. No-rinse shampoos work well for the bedridden patient. They are simply rubbed into the hair and scalp, and no water is needed.

insight

Look beyond the mirror. See the real beauty within.

Foot Care

Foot care is extremely important. The patient's feet should be examined daily, including between the toes and behind the heels.

Symptoms to report:

- Painful or burning feet
- Swollen feet
- Cracks, blisters, cuts or redness
- Changes in skin color or temperature
- Tingling or lack of feeling in the toes or feet

Tips for foot care:

- Do not soak the feet in water unless the doctor prescribes this.
- Do not use any chemicals such as bleach.
- For dry feet, use lotion or cream but do not apply between the toes.
- Cutting corns or calluses can be dangerous. This should only be done by a physician or foot specialist (podiatrist).
- Patients with structural changes of the feet such as hammer-toe, bunions, and contractures should be seen by a podiatrist.
- If the patient's feet are cold, cotton socks can be worn to bed. Cotton is a natural fiber that allows the feet to breathe. Do not use hot water bottles or heating pads to warm the feet.
- Avoid socks or hosiery that bind.
- Shoes should fit properly. Tight or loose shoes can cause blisters.
- Look inside the patient's shoes for small objects, torn linings, and rough areas. These can cause blisters and pain.
- Open-toed shoes or sandals should not be worn unless the

doctor prescribes them.

- The patient should never walk barefoot. It is very easy to stub a toe or cut the foot.
- The patient should avoid sitting with her legs crossed. This puts pressure on the nerves and blood vessels, which can affect circulation to the feet.
- The best shoes are made of breathable natural material, such as leather or canvas.

Nail Care

- Toe nails are softer and easier to cut immediately after bathing.
- Trim the patient's nails as needed, cutting straight across and not down into the corners. Avoid cutting too close to the skin.
- Mineral oil can be used to soften split or cracked nails.
- Smooth sharp nail edges with a nail file.

Summary

In summary, your approach to bathing and other hygiene measures should be with patience and sensitivity. An unclothed person feels especially vulnerable. Therefore, it is important that privacy and respect are considered at all times. By remembering that patient independence is your primary goal when providing care, both you and the patient will benefit.

Chapter 3

Foods & Fluids

Vitamins and minerals obtained from food and fluids are necessary for the body to improve or maintain good health. Many factors may inhibit the patient's ability and desire to eat and drink, which in turn can lead to poor nutrition. Loss of appetite can be an ongoing or temporary problem that requires your patience and encouragement to resolve.

In this chapter you will learn:

- the basics of nutrition and fluid balance
- how to improve the patient's appetite
- how to help the patient eat and drink
- about common digestive problems and special diets

The information about nutrition in this chapter provides general guidelines about the foods you serve the patient. **Any special dietary instructions you receive from medical professionals supersedes this information.**

☞ *Remember:*

YOUR GOAL AS A GOOD CAREGIVER IS TO ALLOW THE PATIENT TO BE AS INDEPENDENT AS HE IS PHYSICALLY AND MENTALLY ABLE TO BE.

Basic Nutrition

Becoming familiar with the six basic food groups will allow you to make wise choices about which foods to prepare and serve. A combination of foods from the various food groups ensures a well-balanced diet that meets the daily requirements of vitamins and minerals. Keep in mind that in many cultures, certain foods and their preparation have symbolic meaning. Do your best to respect the patient's food choices while ensuring adequate nutrition.

Remember, healthful eating is important because it helps the patient

- maintain and improve strength and endurance
- maintain and improve weight
- fight and prevent infection
- heal wounds
- have a feeling of well-being

The Revised Food Pyramid

In April, 2005, the U.S. Department of Agriculture introduced a new food pyramid with more specific advice on portion sizes and calories. The new pyramid contains 6 food categories and also factors in a category for physical exercise.

Grains: Rice, whole grain breads, crackers, cereal, and pasta contain essential nutrients called carbohydrates. They are the major source of energy for the body. Foods in this group also contain fiber, vitamins and minerals.

Vegetables: All vegetables contain carbohydrates, fiber, vitamins and minerals. Serve fresh vegetables instead of canned or frozen whenever possible. Offer them several times a day. Vegetable juice is a tasty, nutritious snack, but watch for sodium content if the patient is on a low sodium diet. Offer a variety of vegetable "colors": dark green, orange, legumes, starchy vegetables.

Fruits: Fruits also contain carbohydrates, fiber, vitamins and minerals. Offer a serving of fruit or fruit juice at each meal or in between meals as a snack. When serving canned or frozen fruit, keep in mind that these often contain added sugar. This may be a concern if the patient is diabetic.

Oils: Most fat should come from sources such as fish, nuts and vegetable oils, limiting solid fats like butter, stick margarine, lard and shortening. Consider using nonstick cooking sprays. They are low in fat and can be substituted for butter and oils for cooking. See the section later in this chapter on Low Cholesterol Diets for additional information.

Milk: Two to three one-cup servings a day from this group can come from foods such as milk, pudding, yogurt, cottage cheese and ice cream. Dairy products are high in protein and calcium, which help keep bones and teeth healthy. They also tend to be high in fat. Consider serving fat-free or low-fat varieties such as skim milk, ice-milk, and low fat yogurt and cottage cheese, if the patient is on a low fat, low cholesterol, or weight reduction diet.

Beans and meat: Lean meat, fish, poultry, eggs, nuts and dry beans contain protein, vitamins and minerals. Protein builds strong muscle, blood, and bone. It helps to heal wounds and increases resistance to infection. Foods from this group should be limited to 1 to 2 four-ounce servings per day. Remove excess fat from meat before cooking and drain grease from meat after browning.

in**sight**

Quality is measured by value, not amount.

Tips for Selecting Healthful Foods

The United States Recommended Daily Allowances (US RDA) are standards developed by the Food and Drug Administration (FDA) for use in regulating nutrition labeling. The nutrition labeling must include the number of calories, and the amount of protein, fat, carbohydrates, and sodium (salt) in a specified serving of a product. It is important to be aware of what a serving size is.

USRDAs for Children Age 4 and Older and for Adults
(Percentages manufacturer must show)

Vitamins and Minerals	100 Percent USRDAs
Vitamin A	1,000 retinol equivalents (RE) or 5,000 International Units (IU)
Vitamin C (ascorbic acid)	60 milligrams (mg)
Thiamine (vitamin B1)	1.5 milligrams (mg)
Riboflavin (vitamin B2)	1.7 milligrams (mg)
Niacin	20 milligrams (mg)
Calcium	1 gram or 1,000 milligrams (mg)
Iron	18 milligrams (mg)

Vitamins and Minerals	100 Percent USRDAs
(Percentages manufacturer may choose to show)	
Vitamin D	400 International Units (IU)
Vitamin E	30 International Units (IU)
Vitamin B6	2 milligrams (mg)
Folic acid (folacin)	0.4 milligrams (mg)
Vitamin B12	6 micrograms (mcg)
Biotin	0.3 milligrams (mg)
Pantothenic acid	10 milligrams (mg)
Phosphorus	1 gram or 1,000 milligrams (mg)
Iodine	150 micrograms (mcg)
Magnesium	400 milligrams (mg)
Zinc	15 milligrams (mg)
Copper	2 milligrams (mg)

- Grocery stores generally carry a variety of health-conscious frozen meals. Check the nutritional information on the labels regarding fat and sodium content before buying.
- Potatoes, pasta, beans, and rice are relatively inexpensive and can be prepared in a variety of ways.
- Many communities have programs that offer well-balanced meals delivered to the patient's home; e.g., Meals on Wheels. Call your local health department for more information about this service.
- Many grocery stores offer delivery services if transportation is an issue. Contact your local supermarket to see if groceries can be ordered through the Internet and delivered to the home.

Fluid Balance

Proper fluid balance must be maintained for good health. Water is lost through perspiration, breathing, and in urine and stools. The amount of fluid that is taken in should equal the amount that is lost. Both food and fluids provide water for the body. Encourage the patient to drink at least 8 eight-ounce glasses of fluid each day, unless the patient's doctor has instructed otherwise.

Facts on Fluids

- Foods that are capable of melting down to a liquid such as pudding, gelatin, sherbet, popsicles and creamed cereals are considered fluids.
- Adequate fluid intake reduces the risk of urinary tract infections and aids in loosening mucous secretions (phlegm).
- The need for additional fluids increases with fever, illness, and hot weather.
- Fever, vomiting and diarrhea can quickly deplete the body of needed fluids resulting in dehydration.

Signs of dehydration:

- decreased or sticky saliva
- decreased urine output
- strong smelling urine
- dryer than normal skin
- absence of tearing in the eyes
- increased confusion

Discuss any concerns about the patient's fluid intake with the doctor.

☞ *Remember:*

THE BEST TREATMENT FOR DEHYDRATION IS PREVENTION.

Loss of Appetite

The patient's appetite and interest in food can change daily. Good nutrition is important, but food should never be forced. If the patient's appetite has decreased, consider that he may be experiencing one or more of the following:

- pain
- sadness, depression, or fear
- fatigue
- anxiety
- nausea
- difficulty swallowing
- mouth sores or ill-fitting dentures

A loss of appetite can also be caused by medications, illness, and chemotherapy.

☞ Remember:

SHORT-TERM LOSS OF APPETITE MAY OCCUR WITH A COLD, MILD FLU, OR FOLLOWING SURGERY. EATING SMALLER AMOUNTS IS ACCEPTABLE AS LONG AS THE PATIENT IS DRINKING PLENTY OF FLUIDS.

Suggestions for Improving Appetite and Nutrition

- Serve six small meals daily instead of three large ones.
- Choose foods high in calories and protein.
- Substitute juices and milkshakes for soda and fruit-flavored beverages.
- Instant potato flakes added to creamed soups and casseroles will boost their nutritional value.
- Adding non-fat dry milk powder to casseroles, meat loaf, mashed potatoes, gravies, creamed soups and cereals increases the calcium and protein content in the food.
- Use a small plate to serve food. A large plate looks overwhelming to someone with a decreased appetite.
- Offer nutritious snacks frequently. Examples of nutritious snacks are dried fruit; blueberry, banana, carrot or bran muffins; fruit juice (not fruit-flavored drinks); vegetable juice; celery or carrot sticks with peanut butter or cream cheese spread; yogurt with fruit, granola or nuts; graham crackers with a glass of milk; hot cereal with honey and raisins.

Commercially prepared liquid food supplements (e.g., Ensure, Boost, Carnation Instant Breakfast) can be offered at mealtime or as a snack. Some contain milk and others are milk free. They are available in a variety of flavors and may be purchased at drug stores, variety stores, and supermarkets.

Be patient during times of appetite loss and don't get discouraged. Do the best you can. But if, despite your efforts, the patient's appetite continues to decline and weight loss is present, consult the doctor.

Helping the Patient Eat and Drink

Knowing when to assist is as important as knowing how to assist. Anything the patient is able to do independently will not only give him a feeling of accomplishment and pride, but will also make your work easier. Keep in mind that the patient's abilities can change from day to day and from meal to meal.

Atmosphere: Provide a comfortable setting. Good companionship during mealtime is beneficial to the patient. Sharing food and conversation is much more enjoyable than eating alone. If the patient wishes to pray before meals, allow adequate time.

Position: Proper positioning is needed for safe and relaxed eating. A patient who is slumped in a wheelchair or whose head is not upright is prone to choking. In bed, raise the head of the bed as high as the patient is able to tolerate. In a wheelchair, position the patient as close to the table as possible. A table that is too high or too low will make eating difficult for the patient.

Feeding Implements: Specially adapted dishes and utensils are widely available, and can enable the patient to eat and drink without help. These can be purchased through a medical supply company, either one in your community or on-line. Occupational therapists specialize in the use of adapted dishes and utensils. Talk to the doctor if you feel this service would benefit the patient.

Cutting and Spreading Board: This implement requires only one hand. It holds bread, toast, crackers or other food items in place while the patient cuts or puts spreads on them.

Plate Guard: This device fits snugly around most ordinary kitchen plates and keeps food from being pushed off the plate.

Adapted Mug: Has two large handles that allow for easy grasp. The lid and spout can be removed. Its wide base helps prevent accidental spills.

Easy Grip Utensils: These utensils work well for the patient with arthritis or limited movement in the hands and fingers. The spoons and forks can be bent to any angle.

When Feeding the Patient

1 Wash your hands.
2 Ensure comfort and good lighting. Have the patient in a sitting position.
3 Protect the patient's clothing with a hand towel, not a bib.
4 Tell the patient what foods you are feeding.
5 Alternate bites of food with sips of liquids.
6 Avoid mixing foods together such as vegetables and fruit.
7 A rubber-coated baby spoon works well for the patient who bites down or is unable to open his mouth wide enough to accommodate a regular utensil.
8 Allow the patient adequate time to chew and swallow each bite of food.
9 Using short straws for drinking requires less energy and effort.
10 Never feed with a syringe. It can easily cause choking.
11 A food processor or blender is an excellent way to puree foods, and costs much less than commercial baby food.
12 Facial grimacing or spitting out food may indicate a dislike for that food.

☞ *Remember:*

FOOD APPEARANCE AND HOW IT IS SERVED AFFECT THE PATIENT'S APPETITE.

Serving the Patient with Poor Vision or Blindness

The "Clock Method" allows the patient who is blind or has poor vision to eat without help. You arrange the food on the plate with the main entree or meat at six o'clock, the vegetable at three o'clock and so on. Be consistent with food placement from meal to meal. Tell the patient what each food item is and where it is located, using numbers as if the plate were a clock; e.g., "Your meat is at six o'clock."

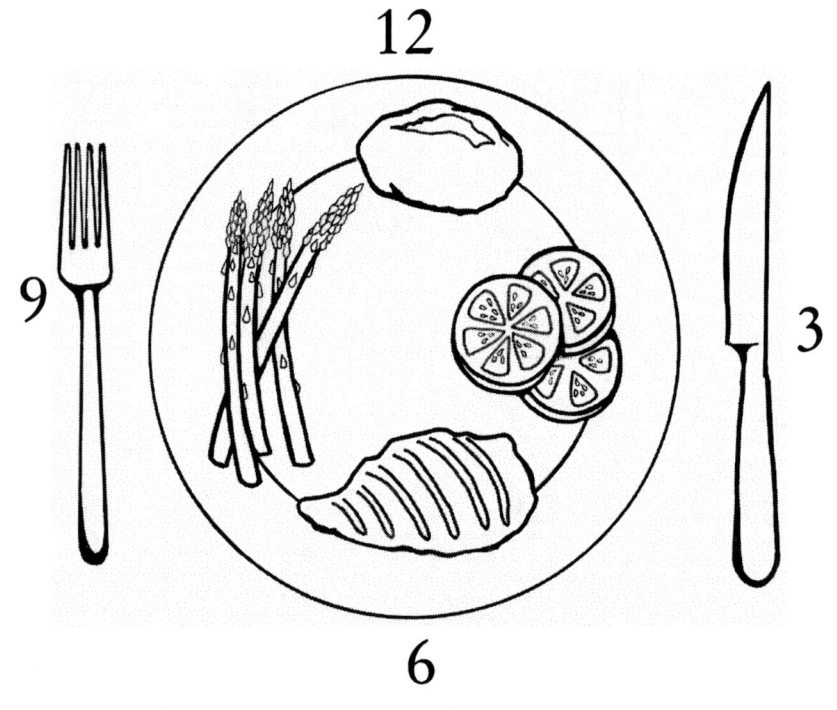

figure 3.1

☞ Remember:

MAKE THE BEST OF TODAY. TOMORROW YOU'LL BE GLAD YOU DID.

Digestive Problems

Nausea, vomiting, diarrhea, and constipation are common digestive problems that can be very distressing to the patient. Diet changes can be made to help lessen the patient's discomfort. If any of these conditions persist, call the doctor.

Vomiting:

- The patient's mouth should be rinsed after vomiting.
- Bright red or coffee ground-colored vomit should be reported to the doctor immediately.
- Offer sips of clear fluids such as apple juice, water, or clear soda when the patient is able to tolerate them.
- Progress to soft/bland foods such as toast, soda crackers, applesauce, bananas, and broth-based soups.
- Resume usual diet after the patient is able to tolerate soft and bland foods.

Nausea:

- Serve fluids 30-60 minutes before or after meals instead of with meals.
- Cool or room temperature foods are better tolerated than warm or hot foods.
- Avoid serving sweet, greasy, and fried foods.

Diarrhea:

- Increase fluids to replace those lost. Avoid apple and pear juice.
- Avoid all milk or milk products, including nutritional supplements containing milk, until the diarrhea has subsided.

- Avoid greasy or spicy foods.
- Avoid gas producing foods such as cauliflower, cabbage and broccoli.
- Encourage low fiber foods such as cooked fruits and vegetables, white bread, pasta, and white rice. Avoid whole grains, such as whole wheat, oats, brown rice, barley, and corn meal. Avoid grapes, prunes, dates, figs, nuts and soft drinks.
- Avoid caffeine (coffee, tea, cola drinks) and chocolate.
- Ask the doctor before giving the patient anti-diarrhea medications. Antacids may worsen diarrhea.

Constipation:
- Serve high fiber foods such as raw fruits and vegetables, whole grain bread and cereal, nuts, and dried fruit.
- Increase fluids to 8 eight-ounce glasses per day. Water is best.
- Offer prunes, prune juice, or apricot nectar one or two times daily.
- Check with the doctor before giving the patient laxatives or stool softeners.

Special Diets

If the patient's doctor has prescribed a special diet, it is important that you know how to select the correct foods. Packaged foods have labels that make it easy to choose the appropriate products. The labels list the ingredients in order from the highest content to the lowest content. The special diets discussed below are a few among many. Additional information on a particular diet can be obtained from the library, Internet, hospital, or doctor's office. There are many cookbooks available that contain wonderful recipes tailored to meet the patient's special diet needs.

Low Salt Diet

(Note: Salt is referred to as "sodium" on food labels.) Too much sodium will cause the body to retain excess fluid, thus increasing the workload of the heart.

- Put the salt shaker away.
- Serve fresh meats, fruits, and vegetables instead of frozen and canned convenience foods.
- Avoid snack foods such as chips, popcorn, crackers, and nuts.
- Avoid bacon, ham, sausage, luncheon meats, and corned beef.
- Catsup, mayonnaise, salad dressings, soy sauce, pickles, olives, seasoning salts, and meat tenderizers should be used sparingly.
- Many foods are available in low salt/sodium varieties. Usually this information is clearly marked on the package label.
- Substitute herbs, spices, and lemon juice for salt.

Low Cholesterol Diet

Cholesterol is a fatty substance found almost exclusively in foods of animal origin. High cholesterol is associated with coronary (heart) artery disease.

- Serve less red meat. Chicken, turkey, venison, veal, and fish should be substituted.
- Ground beef, hot dogs, sausage, bacon, lunch meat, corned beef, organ meats, and shellfish are high in cholesterol and should be avoided.
- Remove skins from chicken and turkey before cooking.
- Avoid all fried foods. Bake or broil foods instead.
- A rack used in the pan when cooking meats will allow the excess fat to drip away from the food.

- Limit dairy products. Avoid those that contain more than 1% milk fat. Check the food labels.
- Avoid nuts, especially cashews, pistachios, and coconut.
- Bakery goods, candy bars, and ice cream should be limited.
- Egg yolks are high in cholesterol. Egg substitutes can be purchased in the refrigerator and frozen food sections of the grocery store.

High Iron Diet

- Good sources of iron are liver, lean red meats, poultry, sesame, pumpkin and sunflower seeds, whole grains, prunes, dried apricots, raisins, legumes, green leafy vegetables, molasses, and cereals fortified with extra iron.
- Include citrus fruits or juices in the same meal that contains iron rich foods. This will boost the iron absorption of those foods. Tea, on the other hand, decreases iron absorption.
- Do not treat the patient's iron deficiency with iron pills unless prescribed by the doctor.

Summary

In summary, nutritious foods and adequate fluids help to keep us healthy. An imbalance of either one can cause malnutrition and dehydration. Temporary loss of appetite is acceptable as long as the patient continues to drink plenty of fluids. There are items available that allow the patient to eat and drink without help. Changing the diet for a short time can lessen the discomforts that are common with digestive problems.

Chapter 4

Waste Elimination

Waste elimination is a normal function of the human body, yet the patient is often embarrassed to discuss this issue with others, including a caregiver. Lack of control over bowel or bladder elimination (incontinence) is devastating. It has a far greater impact on the patient's dignity than you may realize. Incontinence can cause the patient to become isolated and have feelings of low self-esteem.

Caring for a patient who is unable to control urination and bowel movements is one of the most difficult challenges for the caregiver. This challenging job can be accomplished a little bit more easily if you can place yourself in the same situation as the patient. Doing so will help you realize how essential it is to maintain the patient's self-worth when incontinence occurs.

In this chapter you will learn:

- common problems faced with elimination
- solutions to the problems
- skills for catheter care and use of elimination aids
- strategies to reduce urinary incontinence

☞ Remember:

ALLOW THE PATIENT ADEQUATE TIME AND PRIVACY. WASH YOUR HANDS BEFORE AND AFTER USING ELIMINATION AIDS.

Elimination Aids

Commode chair: A commode is a portable toilet that can be placed in any room. It is used by the patient who is able to be out of bed, but unable to get to the bathroom. (figure 4.1)

Bedpan: This plastic container is used for urination and bowel movements when the patient is unable to get out of bed. To use a bedpan, place the patient on her side. Hold the bedpan against the patient's buttocks. Roll the patient back onto the bedpan. Toilet paper and a bell (to call you) should be within reach. When finished, promptly empty the pan into the toilet and flush. Wipe or cleanse the patient as needed. (figure 4.2)

helpful hint:

Powder sprinkled over the edges of the bedpan will help to prevent the bed pan from sticking to the patient's skin.

Urinal: This is a plastic container with a handle that can be used by the male patient to urinate into while lying, sitting, or standing. (figure 4.3)

Raised toilet seat: A plastic seat is used to elevate the height of the toilet making it easier for the patient to transfer on and off the toilet.

Elimination aids can be purchased or rented at medical supply stores.

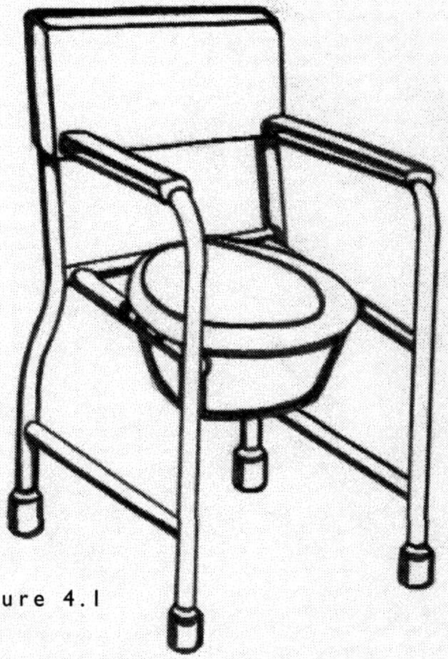

figure 4.1

figure 4.2

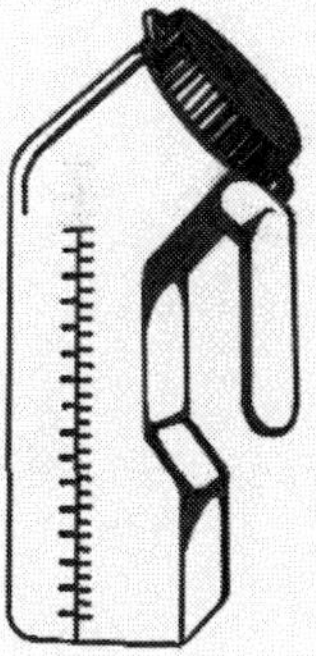

figure 4.3

Remember:

URINE OR STOOL FROM COMMODES, BEDPANS, AND URINALS SHOULD BE PROMPTLY EMPTIED AND FLUSHED DOWN THE TOILET. CLEANSE THE CONTAINERS AFTER EACH USE WITH LIQUID SOAP AND HOT WATER, FOLLOWED BY A HOUSEHOLD DISINFECTANT, SUCH AS LYSOL™ OR BLEACH. RINSE THE DEVICE AND DRY WELL.

Normal Bowel Movements

The frequency of bowel movements varies from patient to patient, ranging from two to three movements per day to one or two per week. It is important to watch for sudden changes

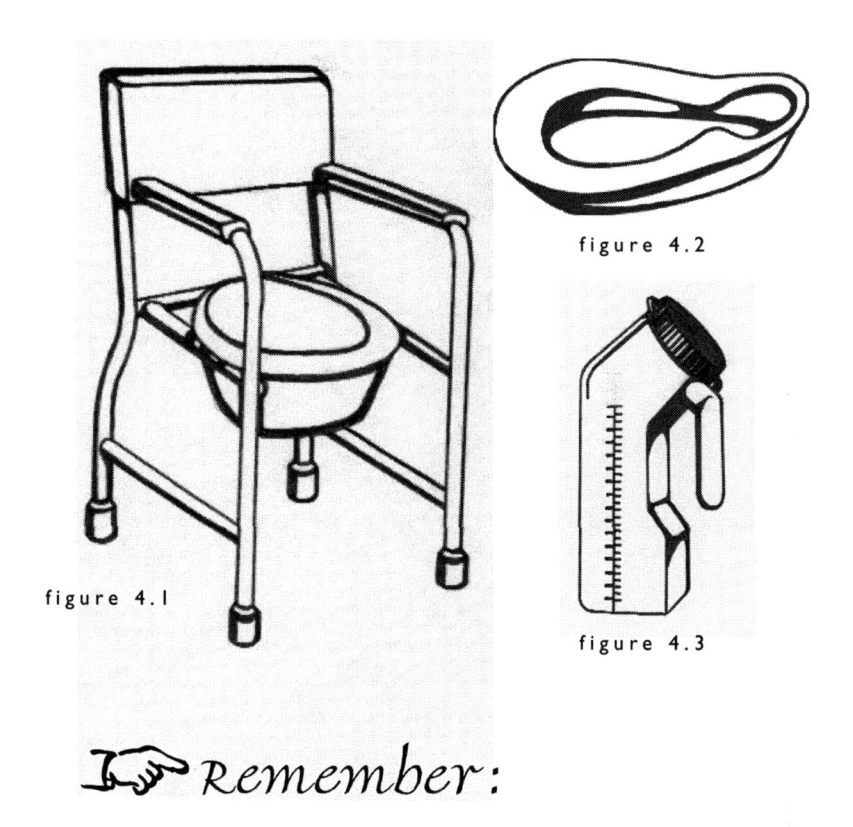

in bowel habits. If the patient normally has a bowel movement every day and then doesn't have one for four days, that is a significant change in bowel habits. It is not necessary that the patient have a bowel movement every day if her normal pattern is every third day

A normal stool is brown, soft, moist, and formed. Bowel movements should occur easily and painlessly. If the patient is able, a bathroom toilet or commode should be used instead of a bedpan.

Common Problems

Constipation, diarrhea, hemorrhoids, and bowel incontinence can disrupt the patient's daily activities. Becoming aware of the possible causes can prevent these problems from occurring.

Constipation

Constipation is defined as stools that are hard, dry, and difficult to pass. The patient may strain to have a bowel movement, or complain of pressure and fullness in the rectum or lower abdomen.

Possible causes of constipation are:

- too little fiber in foods
- inadequate fluid intake
- overeating or inadequate chewing
- too little exercise
- depression, stress, anxiety
- tight-fitting clothing
- poor posture
- iron supplements, pain medications
- abuse of laxatives
- ignoring the urge to have a bowel movement
- change in routine

helpful hint:

If the patient drinks one to two cups of warm water each morning before breakfast, this will help to soften the stools. *See page 35 for dietary advice.*

Remember:

STOOL SOFTENERS, LAXATIVES, OR SUPPOSITORIES SHOULD BE ADMINISTERED ONLY WITH THE DOCTOR'S APPROVAL.

To insert a suppository:

- Wash your hands.
- Place a waterproof pad or bath towel under the patient's buttocks.
- Have the patient lie on her left side, if possible.
- Wear disposable gloves. Apply a generous amount of lubrication (water soluble) to the suppository. Do not use petroleum jelly. Ask the pharmacist for the proper lubrication.
- For best results, insert the suppository along the wall of the rectum as high as your finger can reach.
- Remove and dispose of the gloves immediately and wash your hands.
- Suppositories must be stored in the refrigerator to keep them from melting.

Diarrhea

Diarrhea is defined as the urgent and frequent passage of unformed watery stools (more than three per day). It may be accompanied by abdominal cramping, nausea, and vomiting.

Possible causes of diarrhea are:

- infection or illness
- food allergy, or a side effect of medication, such as an antibiotic
- intolerance to greasy or spicy foods
- abuse of laxatives
- stress, anxiety

The patient's anal area should be cleansed and dried after each watery bowel movement. Apply a protective ointment to the area, such as Vaseline™ or A&D™. This will help to prevent skin breakdown and irritation. Talk with the doctor before giving anti-diarrheal medications. See page 34 for dietary advice.

☞ *Remember:*

WASH YOUR HANDS BEFORE AND AFTER HANDLING URINE OR STOOL. DON'T FORGET TO WEAR DISPOSABLE GLOVES.

Hemorrhoids

Hemorrhoids are enlarged blood vessels present inside or outside the rectum or anus. They can cause itching and pain. Bleeding may occur with bowel movements.

Possible causes of hemorrhoids are:

- straining with bowel movements
- constipation
- prolonged sitting

The treatment for hemorrhoids varies from a topical ointment, such as Preparation H™, and a cool compress, such as a

Tucks™ pad, to a surgical procedure. The doctor will decide which treatment is best for the patient.

Bowel Incontinence

Bowel incontinence is the involuntary passage of stool.

Possible causes of bowel incontinence are:

- depression, severe anxiety
- inadequate relaxation
- multiple life changes
- poor nutrition
- little or no exercise
- physical problems with the bones, muscles, or nervous system
- confusion or dementia, such as Alzheimer's

Provide the bedpan or commode to the patient after meals and every two to three hours. Good skin care is required following each bowel movement.

When to Call the Doctor

- If there is a sudden change in the frequency of bowel movements.
- If the patient suddenly is unable to control her bowel movements. This may be a sign of an impaction, which is a hard or pasty accumulation of stool that the patient is unable to pass.
- If the stools are black, tarry, or contain blood.
- If there is abdominal bloating and pain.
- If weight loss and fatigue are present.
- If constipation or diarrhea frequently recurs.
- If the medications the doctor has prescribed aren't working.
- If hemorrhoids are suspected.

insight

Draw from your past experiences and you will find great strength in your abilities.

Normal Urination

Urination or "voiding" is the process of emptying the bladder. It should occur without effort or pain. Normal urine is clear and pale yellow or amber in color. How much the patient urinates will depend on many factors such as fluid intake, perspiration, vomiting, diarrhea, and medications. The average person urinates five to six times a day and occasionally once at night. Observe the patient's usual pattern of urination. Be alert to any changes.

Urinary Incontinence

Urinary incontinence is the inability to hold urine in the bladder long enough to get to a toilet. Incontinence can be a symptom of underlying problems. It is often left untreated because the patient or caregiver is unsure of how to manage the incontinence. The doctor can advise you on the best way to manage and treat the patient's condition.

Possible causes of incontinence are:

- damage to the nervous system, such as stroke, paralysis, or confusion
- infection (see page 49 for symptoms of urinary tract infections)
- muscle weakness in the area that controls urination
- limited ability to move

- illness
- clothing that is difficult for the patient to remove
- obesity, which can weaken the pelvic muscles

☞ Remember:

URINARY INCONTINENCE CAN BE HUMILIATING AND DISTRESSING TO THE PATIENT. EVERYTHING SHOULD BE DONE TO MANAGE THE INCONTINENCE WHILE PRESERVING THE PATIENT'S DIGNITY AND SELF-ESTEEM.

Stress Incontinence

The muscles that control the release of urine can become weakened, and urination can occur while coughing, sneezing, laughing, or with mild exercise. Stress incontinence may decrease with exercise that strengthens muscle tone.

Exercises to Strengthen Muscle Tone (Kegal Exercises) for Men and Women

While the patient is urinating, ask her to try to stop the urine flow. Repeat several times. After the patient learns to recognize what muscles are used to control urine flow, she can practice tightening these same muscles at any time, place, or position. By strengthening the muscles that control urination, the patient's ability to hold urine in the bladder will improve.

Catheters

A catheter is a rubber or plastic tube that drains urine from the bladder into a collecting bag. Catheters are needed for many reasons such as incontinence, bladder problems, or following surgery. Whatever the reason, special care is needed to keep the catheter tubing and insertion site clean. Good hygiene helps to minimize the risk of infection. The area around the catheter, as well as the genital area, should be washed, rinsed, and dried twice a day, and more often if necessary. The patient's catheter bag should always hang at a level below the patient's bladder, to keep the urine from returning to the bladder. Do not allow the catheter bag to touch the floor. Drain the urine from the catheter bag every four to six hours or when it becomes two-thirds full.

☞ Remember:

USE DISPOSABLE GLOVES AND A CLEAN WASHCLOTH EACH TIME YOU DO CATHETER CARE.

When emptying a catheter bag:

1 Wash your hands.
2 Wear disposable gloves.
3 Place a paper towel on the floor below the catheter bag.
4 Place a container that will only be used to collect urine on the paper towel. Drain the urine into the container.
5 Before closing the release mechanism at the bottom of the catheter bag, clean it with rubbing alcohol and a cotton ball.
6 Observe the urine for abnormalities in color and amount. Look in both the bag and the tubing.
7 Empty the urine into the toilet and flush. Remove the gloves and dispose of them. Wash your hands.
8 Check the tubing to make sure it is free of any kinks that could interfere with urine flow.

Incontinence Aids and Products

There are a wide variety of aids to help with incontinence problems, whether bowel- or bladder-related.

- An alarm clock can be helpful in reminding the patient to use the bathroom.
- Incontinence pads and pants such as Dry Pride™, Depends™, or Serenity™ are made of absorbent material and work on the same principle as a diaper. They fit inside the patient's underwear, or are worn instead of underwear.
- A waterproof protector fits over the mattress like a fitted sheet to protect the bedding. A regular fitted sheet is placed over it. Waterproof protectors can be purchased at variety stores and large department stores.
- An absorbent bed pad can be placed directly under the patient to absorb wetness and protect the bedding. Bed pads can be purchased at medical supply stores.

Using Incontinence Products

Reassuring the patient that urinary incontinence is a common, manageable problem in older adults will help to eliminate some of the fear, anxiety, and embarrassment associated with the use of incontinence products.

What incontinence products do:

- Absorb and prevent leakage onto clothing, bedding, and furniture
- Control odor and are comfortable to wear
- Protect the skin from breaking down with painful chafing and pressure sores
- Easily disposed of
- Are unnoticeable under clothing
- Reasonably priced and readily available at grocery stores, variety stores, and drug stores

Incontinence products are offered in a variety of absorbencies, from thin pads to full briefs. Choosing the most appropriate product will depend on the amount of absorbency needed.

Strategies to Reduce Urinary Incontinence

Many of these strategies are used effectively with patients who have Alzheimer's disease. However, the degree to which the patient responds will depend on the level of dementia and her ability to understand and comprehend.

1 Scheduled toileting: Set up a routine voiding schedule. Have the patient use the toilet, urinal, or bedpan every 2 to 3 hours.
2 Prompted voiding: Encourage the patient to use the toilet at regular intervals. Give praise for maintaining continence.
3 Visual cues: Label the bathroom with easy-to-read signs or pictures. Leave a nightlight on at night to draw the patient's attention to the bathroom.
4 Simplified clothing: Clothing with elastic waistbands and Velcro™ strips (to replace buttons and zippers) can be removed quickly and easily, thus reducing the anxiety of getting to the bathroom on time.
5 Verbal coaching: Cueing is effective for the patient who does not remember how to get started in the task of using the bathroom, but when coached can complete the task.

helpful hint:

Diuretics (water pills) increase the amount of urine excreted from the body. Diuretics given during the day will decrease the chances that incontinence will occur during the night.

☞ Remember:

DO NOT RESTRICT THE PATIENT'S FLUIDS IN AN EFFORT TO REDUCE URINARY INCONTINENCE. THIS PRACTICE CAN LEAD TO DEHYDRATION.

Urinary Tract Infection

The patient may develop an infection in the kidneys (which produce urine); in the bladder (which holds the urine); or in the urethra (which is the tube that drains the urine to the outside of the body). By learning to recognize, treat, and prevent urinary tract infections, hospitalization can often be prevented.

Symptoms of urinary tract infection:

- fever, vomiting
- pain or burning with urination
- frequent or urgent need to urinate
- urine that is cloudy, dark, contains blood, or has an unusually strong odor
- dribbling or voiding unusually small amounts at a time
- pain in the lower back or lower abdomen

If the patient is showing some of the signs that a urinary tract infection may be present, call the doctor's office. The doctor may want a sample of urine from the patient to be tested for infection.

Collecting a Urine Sample

1 Wash your hands before and after collecting the urine sample. Wear disposable gloves.

2 A sterile cup or container should be used if the patient is able to sit on a toilet or commode. A sterile cup can be obtained from the doctor's office or clinical laboratory. If the patient is bedridden, ask the doctor's office for specific instructions on collecting the urine sample.
3 Wash and rinse the patient's genital area well before collecting the urine sample.
4 Have the patient urinate a small amount into the toilet, then quickly position the specimen cup near, but not touching the patient. Collect at least one ounce (six teaspoons) into the cup.
5 Put the lid onto the cup immediately. Avoid touching the inside of the container or lid.
6 Dispose of the gloves, and wash your hands.
7 Refrigerate the urine. Take the specimen to the doctor's office or laboratory as soon as possible.

Treating a Urinary Tract Infection

- The doctor may prescribe an antibiotic to treat the infection.
- The patient should take the medication until it is completely finished.
- Give the medication at evenly spaced times as the doctor or pharmacist has instructed. Do not miss doses.
- Call the doctor if the patient develops a rash or any other unusual symptom while taking the medication. The pharmacist will advise you on what side effects to watch for, as each medication is different.
- If the patient's symptoms are still present, or if they return after the medication has been finished, notify the doctor.

Preventing a Urinary Tract Infection

- Ensure that good hygiene is maintained.
- Encourage fluids, at least eight to ten glasses of water a day, in addition to fruit juices such as orange, grapefruit, or cranberry.
- Have the patient urinate as soon as she feels the need. Holding the urine back only allows the germs more time to multiply.
- Use pure soaps that are free of dyes, perfumes, and deodorants, such as Ivory or Dove. Soaps that contain dyes, perfumes, and deodorants can irritate the patient's skin which can lead to infection.
- If possible, have the patient shower instead of bathing in the tub. Sitting in bath water allows germs to work their way into the patient's urinary tract.
- Try to prevent constipation. It can contribute to urinary tract infections.

Reminders:

For women:

- Always wipe from front to back after urinating.
- Cotton underwear should be worn.
- Urinate immediately after intercourse.
- Toilet paper should be white and free of perfumes.

For men:

- Problems with the prostate gland can affect urination. Notify the doctor if the patient is having difficulty in starting the urine stream, or if the stream is very slow and narrow.

Skin Breakdown

- Urine soaked clothing can cause the skin to become reddened and painful. Sores can quickly develop. Promptly change the patient's wet clothing and bedding.
- Every time incontinence occurs, wash the urine from the skin with mild soap and warm water. Rinse and pat dry.
- Barrier creams or ointments, such as Vaseline, Desitin, and A&D, can be used to help keep urine away from the skin. They can be purchased at drug stores or variety stores. A pharmacist can assist you in selecting the best product for the patient.

in**sight**

Each phase of your life will bring new challenges and joy.

Summary

In summary, loss of control over the bowels and bladder is extremely distressing to the patient. Always seek medical advice from the patient's doctor for her bowel and bladder problems. There are solutions to allow the patient to regain independence, such as elimination aids. Prevention of common problems, such as diarrhea and constipation, can significantly improve the patient's well being. Recognizing early signs and symptoms of a urinary tract infection can facilitate quick recovery. With attentive care and a watchful eye, you can significantly improve the patient's quality of life.

Chapter 5

Mobility

Mobility is the ability to move around from place to place and from sitting to standing. Most of us take mobility for granted when we are healthy. Little thought is given to caring for the muscles and the bones that support healthy movement.

Illness or injury involving any body system can interfere with the patient's ability to move. This added fatigue and stress can be so overwhelming that even the thought of moving around is distressing to the patient. As the caregiver, you have the potential to exert the greatest influence on the patient, so that he may achieve optimum physical strength and mobility.

In this chapter, you will learn

- what factors affect the patient's ability to walk
- instructions for simple exercises that will improve the patient's overall well-being
- why adequate rest is important for the patient
- tips on helping the patient move from a bed to a chair
- helpful assistive devices that will encourage independence and make mobility achievable

Remember:

BEING DEPENDENT ON ANOTHER PERSON MAY BE A GREAT CONCERN TO THE PATIENT. IT IS VERY IMPORTANT THAT YOU ALLOW HIM TO PERFORM EVEN THE SIMPLEST OF TASKS IN ORDER TO FOSTER A SENSE OF INDEPENDENCE.

Exercise

Encouraging exercise is one of the most important things you can do for the patient. You may have to provide instructions and monitor the patient to ensure that the exercises are done properly.

The patient will enjoy the responsibility and independence that comes from performing his own exercises *(active exercise)*. If the patient is unable to exercise independently, it will be up to you to exercise his muscles and joints for him *(passive exercise)*. Exercise can improve the patient's quality of life, which will have a significant impact on his productivity.

If the patient's doctor has ordered a physical or occupational therapist's services, prepare the home and the patient by:

- ensuring walkways are clear and free of clutter
- removing throw rugs
- providing ample lighting
- administering pain medication (if ordered by the doctor) 30 to 60 minutes prior to the therapist's visit
- having the patient toileted and in comfortable clothing
- ensuring that the patient is wearing well-fitting shoes with non-skid soles

See Chapter 11 for more information on physical and occupational therapy.

Some guidelines to follow for active or passive exercise:

- Never exercise a swollen, reddened joint.
- Never exercise beyond the point of pain.
- Never exercise to the point of fatigue.

- Stop exercising immediately if the patient complains of:
  - chest pain
  - dizziness
  - blurred vision
  - shortness of breath
  - pain in the neck, jaw, or arms

insight

Strength is measured not by our bodies, but by our souls.

Active and Passive Exercise

Both active and passive exercise will improve the patient's ability to move his joints and will increase circulation to the exercised parts. In order for the patient to increase muscle mass and strength, the exercises must be performed by the patient.

Give simple instructions while demonstrating each exercise. The patient will be more eager to exercise on a regular basis if you participate with him. Lively music can make exercising fun.

Active exercise can be performed by the patient in different positions. Passive exercises are accomplished best if the patient is lying on his back. Each movement should be repeated five to ten times, on each side of the body, or as the patient is able to tolerate. Exercises should be performed two to three times a day. Properly performing these exercises is as important as spending adequate time to complete each one.

Head

1 Turn the head to the right, and then to the left.
2 Move the right ear toward the right shoulder. Return to starting position. Move the left ear toward the left shoulder. Return to starting position.

Shoulder

1 With the elbow straight and along side of the body, raise the arm up towards the head. Lower the arm to starting position.
2 With the elbow straight and the arm away from the body, raise the arm up towards the head. Return to starting position.

Elbow

1 Bend the arm at the elbow and straighten again.
2 Extend the arm outward to shoulder level. Sweep the arm across the chest toward the opposite shoulder. Return to starting position.

Wrists

With the elbow bent, bend the wrist up, down, and from side to side.

Hand and Fingers

1 Make a fist, then straighten the fingers.
2 Spread the fingers apart, then bring them back together.

Hip

1 In a seated position, keeping the knee straight, lift one leg up as high as possible. Return to starting position.
2 Gently move the leg out to one side. Return to starting position.
3 With the legs straight, turn both knees inward, then turn both knees away from each other. Return to starting position

Knee
In a seated position, while bending the knee, bring it up towards the chest. Straighten the knee as you lower the leg back down.

Ankle
1 Point the toes toward the knees, then point the toes toward the ground.
2 Move the ankle to the left and then to the right.

Toes
Bend the toes down and then straighten them.

☞ Remember:

ACTIVITIES, SUCH AS WORKING PUZZLES, FOLDING CLOTHES, AND WRITING, EXERCISE THE JOINTS AND SHOULD BE ENCOURAGED.

Assistive Devices

Assistive devices are aids that can greatly improve the patient's ability to move. They make difficult tasks easier and safer. To insure that assistive devices are the proper height and fit, they should be measured and fitted by a trained professional, such as a physical therapist. Medical supply stores generally offer this service. All listed assistive devices can be purchased at medical supply stores. Ask about used equipment or rentals as an option. You may also be able to borrow assistive devices from a local hospital, through Hospice, or from charitable organizations.

Transfer Belt

A transfer or gait belt is a wide belt that is placed snugly around the patient's waist. By holding on to the transfer belt, a caregiver has better control when assisting the patient with ambulation or transfers. Always put a transfer belt on the outside of the patient's clothing or pajamas, never immediately next to the skin.

Walkers

Walkers provide firm support and offer security to an unsteady patient. They are available with or without front wheels. Walkers with front wheels are best for the patient who is unable to lift the walker. Many can be folded into a compact position for ease in travel. Make sure that the rubber tips on the legs of the walker are in good condition.

Cane

Canes are available with curved or straight handles. Some have three- or four-pronged legs that provide a wide base of support for the patient. The handle of a cane should be level with the patient's wrist when his arm is hanging at his side. Remind the patient not to lean out over the cane.

Stair Lift

A stair lift is a mechanical chair that is attached to the staircase. The patient simply sits in the chair, pushes a button, and it slowly moves up or down the staircase. A stair lift is an excellent device for the patient who has difficulty getting up and down the stairs.

Crutches

Crutches offer more support than a cane and can be used singly or in pairs. Crutches may be used to help strengthen the legs, or in situations where the use of a leg is to be avoided.

Wheelchairs

There are a wide variety of wheelchairs available, depending on the patient's specific needs. They range from self-propelled to power-driven. Wheelchairs can be adapted to improve comfort and positioning. A doctor or physical therapist can advise you on the type of wheelchair that would most benefit the patient.

Mechanical Lift

A mechanical lift is a battery-operated piece of equipment used to safely transfer a patient who is unable to bear weight or when the caregiver is unable to comfortably transfer him using other transfer methods. A mechanical lift is ideal for a patient who is very heavy or whose physical stature makes safe transfers and maneuvers difficult. A Pal type mechanical lift works well for the patient who can bear weight but is unable to transfer safely. Mechanical lifts eliminate the risk of back injury for the caregiver.

Mobility Scooter

Medical electric scooters have either three or four wheels and steer much like a bicycle, using handlebars. Electric scooters are ideal for out-of-home activities, as they glide smoothly and easily over a variety of surfaces. There are even portable motorized scooters that can be stowed in the trunk of your car to take along with you.

Walking With or Without Help

Walking, or moving about in an upright position, is known as ambulation. Walking is an excellent form of exercise, and improves overall body functioning. Walking with or without help requires both strength and balance. Promote and encourage walking several times a day, if the patient is able.

Benefits of Ambulation

- Strengthens muscles, moves joints
- Stimulates circulation
- Decreases the risk of skin breakdown
- Stimulates the bowels
- Decreases the risk of urinary tract infection
- Improves digestion of foods
- Increases lung expansion which helps decrease the risk of respiratory infections, such as pneumonia
- Promotes a positive self-image
- Provides a feeling of independence

Factors Adversely Affecting Ambulation

- Poor vision
- Loss of coordination, dizziness
- Weakness, pain
- Illness or injury

The patient who is able to walk unassisted should be allowed to do so, but remember that his ability can change from day to day. He may be reluctant to ask for your help. Focus on the patient's existing abilities and assist him as needed.

☞ Remember:

THE PATIENT WHO IS WEAK OR UNSTEADY ON HIS FEET IS AT RISK FOR FALLS. INTERVENE, IF YOU FEEL THE PATIENT'S SAFETY IS JEOPARDIZED.

Assisting with Ambulation

When assisting the patient with ambulating, his safety—as well as your own—must be considered. Your goal as the caregiver is to maintain or improve the patient's mobility level, while at the same time avoiding falls and injury.

Some tips for assisting:

- If the patient has a walker or cane for ambulation, encourage him to use it instead of relying on furniture for support and balance.
- Clear the pathway of hazards that could cause tripping.
- Assist the patient to a sitting position first. This allows him time to gain balance.
- Put the patient's shoes on.
- Apply a transfer belt around the patient's waist. (See page 58 for information on transfer belts.)
- Grab the transfer belt with both hands, one hand on each side of the patient.
- Slowly assist the patient to a standing position while you stand directly in front of him, or on his weaker side.
- Allow the patient to stand for a minute or two to gain his balance before beginning to ambulate.
- Encourage good posture (standing upright with his head and back erect).
- Walk behind and slightly to the side of the patient while continuing to hold onto the transfer belt. Hold the belt with one hand at the back and one hand at the side of the patient. (figure 5.1)

- Instruct the patient to lift his feet when walking. Dragging the feet increases the risk of falling.
- Allow the patient to ambulate at a safe and comfortable pace.
- Ambulate only as far as the patient is able to tolerate. Increase the distance gradually.
- Instruct the patient to take deep breaths while walking. This promotes good intake of oxygen and lung expansion.

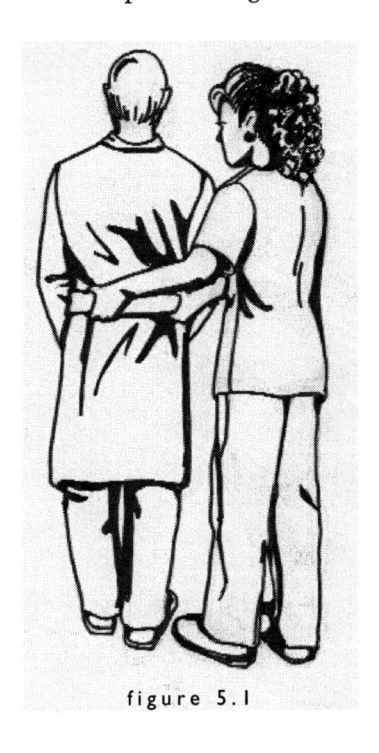

figure 5.1

Remember:

LENGTHY PERIODS OF BED REST ARE NOT NECESSARY DURING MOST ILLNESSES OR FOLLOWING SURGERY. THE PATIENT NEEDS TO BE UP AND WALKING UNLESS THE DOCTOR HAS SPECIFIED OTHERWISE.

Transferring

Transferring is the act of moving the patient from one position to another position in a different place. An example would be moving a patient from the bed to a wheel chair. Sometimes moving from a bed to a chair takes a significant amount of the patient's energy. Care must be taken to help him maintain good posture and protect him from injury while you help with transfers. Know the patient's capabilities and ask the doctor about any movement that is not allowed.

Guidelines for Transfers

- Plan what you will do before you attempt to help with transfers. Tell the patient what that plan is.
- Remove any obstacles from the needed pathways.
- If the patient wears braces or body supports, put these on first before helping him out of bed.
- Allow the patient to use whatever strength he has to help. This will lessen your work.

The following techniques do not involve any lifting. We will explain how to move the patient by transferring body weight. The risk of injury to yourself (especially back strain) or to the patient is increased if you transfer incorrectly. Make sure that these procedures are demonstrated to you by the doctor, a registered nurse, or an occupational or physical therapist before you attempt to transfer the patient on your own. *(See page 117 for more information regarding physical and occupational therapy.)*

Transferring from a bed to a chair (can be a wheelchair or commode):

- Tell the patient what you plan to do.
- Put non-skid shoes on the patient.
- Position the chair beside the bed on the patient's strongest side.
- Swing back or remove the wheelchair foot rests (if this applies).
- Lock the wheels of the bed and wheelchair.
- Make sure the bed is in the lowest position and the side rail is down, if this applies.
- Help the patient to a sitting position on the side of the bed. Allow him to remain sitting in this position for a few minutes. This will allow his body time to adjust to a change of position.
- Apply a transfer belt around the patient's waist. (See page 58 for information on transfer belts.) Grip the transfer belt at the sides of his waist with one hand on each side.
- Assist the patient to the edge of the bed until his feet are resting on the floor.
- Stand directly in front of the patient. He should put his hands on your shoulders or on the arms of the chair, if able.
- Brace your legs and knees against his. Keep your feet about eighteen inches apart for better balance.
- Help the patient into position directly in front of the chair. This ensures that the patient is properly positioned before sitting.
- Gently assist the patient into a sitting position.
- Remove the transfer belt.

☞ *Remember:*

BEND AT YOUR KNEES, NOT AT YOUR WAIST, WHEN HELPING WITH TRANSFERS.

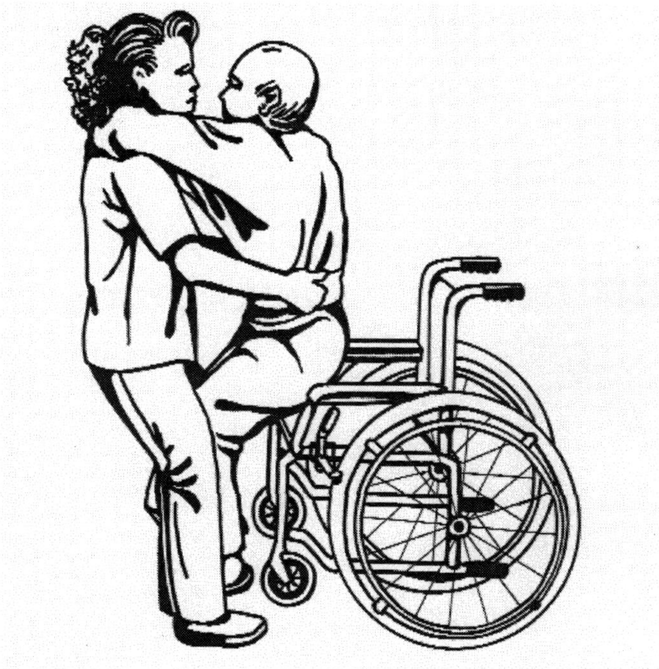

figure 5.2

Transferring from a chair to a bed:

- Apply a transfer belt around the patient's waist. *(See page 58 for information on transfer belts.)*
- Lock the wheels of the bed and wheelchair.
- Help the patient move to the edge of the chair.
- Stand in front of the patient with your knees against the outside of his knees. Keep your feet about eighteen inches apart.
- Tell the patient to put his hands on your shoulders while you bend at the knees.
- Grip the transfer belt at each side of the patient's waist.
- With a rocking motion, ask the patient to stand up on the count of three. As the patient stands, straighten your back and knees.

- Assist the patient to pivot so that the back of his legs are touching the bed.
- Lower the patient to a sitting position.
- Remove the transfer belt.

insight

Small steps forward will lead to giant strides.

Rest

While the effects of exercise are extremely beneficial, it is important that the patient have adequate rest. The patient should have a balance of activity and rest periods.

Benefits of Rest

- Restores a feeling of well-being
- Relieves stress and anxiety
- Improves coping ability
- Improves the ability to concentrate on activities of daily living

Summary

In summary, the patient's mobility level has an impact on his ability to perform activities of daily living. Your efforts to maintain or improve this level will benefit both you and the patient. Keeping the patient's muscles and joints exercised will improve his overall well-being. Assistive devices are available to enable the patient to reach his optimum capabilities.

Chapter 6

Caregiver Skills

There are times when you will be called upon to check the patient's vital signs and provide a report to her doctor or nurse. Once you are familiar with the patient's usual or "normal" vital signs, you will be able to recognize a significant change.

In this chapter you will learn

- how to monitor the patient's temperature, pulse, and respiration (vital signs)
- how to monitor and administer medications safely
- when to use heat and cold applications

With basic knowledge, practice, and faith in your abilities, you will be successful in learning these important skills.

Temperature

Body temperature is the amount of heat in the body. It is a balance between the amount of heat produced by the body and the amount of heat lost. If this balance is disturbed, a body temperature that is abnormally high or low will result. A normal body temperature is between 96.8 degrees Fahrenheit (36.0 Celsius) and 98.6 degrees Fahrenheit (37.0 Celsius). Temperatures above or below this range should be reported to the patient's doctor. An abnormal temperature is often a sign of illness.

Factors that increase body temperature:

- infection or illness
- dehydration
- hot weather
- warm blankets or heavy clothing
- physical activity and exercise

Factors that decrease body temperature:

- shock (decreased circulation)
- cold weather
- medications, such as aspirin, acetaminophen (e.g.,Tylenol™), or ibuprofen (e.g., Motrin™)
- age (older people tend to have a lower "normal" body temperature)

Signs of a high body temperature (fever)	Signs of a low body temperature
shivering or chills	cool-feeling skin
sweating (perspiring)	pale-looking skin
skin that feels hot	shivering
flushed cheeks or face	complaints of feeling cold
complaints of feeling warm or hot	unusual confusion

Taking a Temperature

Two common methods for obtaining the patient's temperature are orally (by mouth) and axillary (under the armpit). Thermometers are made of either glass (mercury) or plastic (digital). Regardless of the method you choose, certain guidelines must be followed.

- Wash your hands before and after handling a thermometer.
- Glass or plastic thermometers should be wiped off with rubbing alcohol before and after each use.
- You must shake down the mercury on a glass thermometer to the bottom of the scale before using it.
- Never use a thermometer that is cracked or chipped.
- Oral/axillary glass thermometers have a blue-end tip.

Remember:

IF THE PATIENT HAS HAD HOT OR COLD BEVERAGES, OR HAS SMOKED A CIGARETTE, WAIT 30 MINUTES BEFORE TAKING AN ORAL TEMPERATURE TO ENSURE AN ACCURATE READING.

Taking an Oral Temperature

Using a glass thermometer:

1. Place the thermometer under the patient's tongue. Ask her to close her mouth and lips securely around the thermometer
2. Leave the thermometer in the patient's mouth for 3 to 5 minutes
3. Remove the thermometer and record the temperature.4. Shake the mercury back down. Clean the thermometer with alcohol and return it to its case

Using a plastic (digital) thermometer:

1. Turn the thermometer on. Wait until a blank screen appears
2. Place the thermometer under the patient's tongue. Ask her to close her mouth and lips securely around the thermometer
3. Remove the thermometer after you hear it beep. Record the temperature

4. Turn the thermometer off. Clean the thermometer with alcohol and return it to its case

Do not take an oral temperature if the patient

- has had head or neck surgery, or has suffered an injury anywhere on the face or neck
- breathes through her mouth, has a cough, or a stuffy, blocked nose
- has a sore mouth
- has a history of convulsions or seizures
- is restless, disoriented, or confused

Taking an Axillary Temperature

1. Place the thermometer under the patient's armpit. Make sure the armpit is dry
2. The thermometer bulb (tip) must be in full contact with the patient's skin. The patient's arm should rest along her side, or across her chest
3. If you are using a glass thermometer, leave it in place for a full 5 minutes
4. If you are using a digital thermometer, leave it in place until you hear it beep
5. Record the temperature. Clean the thermometer with alcohol, then return it to its case
6. An axillary temperature is usually a degree lower than a temperature taken orally

Remember:

DO NOT TAKE THE PATIENT'S TEMPERATURE RECTALLY. COMPLICATIONS CAN OCCUR.

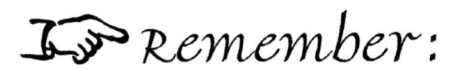

Taking a Temperature via the Ear

A tympanic thermometer may be used to take the patient's temperature via the ear canal. A tympanic thermometer can obtain a temperature in seconds. Mercury, digital, and tympanic thermometers can be purchased at drug stores and variety stores. All thermometers come with detailed instructions on their use.

Comfort Measures for a High Temperature

Your goal is to lower the patient's temperature, which will make her more comfortable. Call the doctor with all temperature concerns. The following are general guidelines for lowering a high temperature. In all cases, the doctor's or nurse's specific directions for the patient should be followed.

- Fever-reducing medications such as acetaminophen (Tylenol™) or ibuprofen (Motrin™) will reduce the discomforts caused by a high temperature. Check with the doctor before administering either
- Apply a cool washcloth to the patient's forehead or the back of her neck
- Sponge the patient's body with cool water. Pat her skin dry to avoid chilling
- If the patient is perspiring, change her clothing and bedding as needed
- Offer frequent cold drinks or popsicles
- Provide adequate room ventilation. A fan may be used on a low setting, but do not aim it directly at the patient
- Dress the patient in lightweight clothing and remove all heavy blankets

Comfort Measures for a Low Temperature

The patients at greatest risk for developing a low body temperature are the frail, ill, elderly, and immobile. Again, these are general guidelines for providing comfort to the patient with a low temperature.

- Keep the room temperature warm. Remember that nights get cooler (figure 6.1 on previous page)
- Offer warm foods and frequent warm drinks
- Encourage increased activity (movement and exercise)
- Dress the patient in several layers of light clothing. This is more effective than one thick layer

Pulse

Taking the patient's pulse is a simple way to determine how fast or slow her heart is beating. In an adult, a normal pulse rate is between 60 and 100 beats per minute.

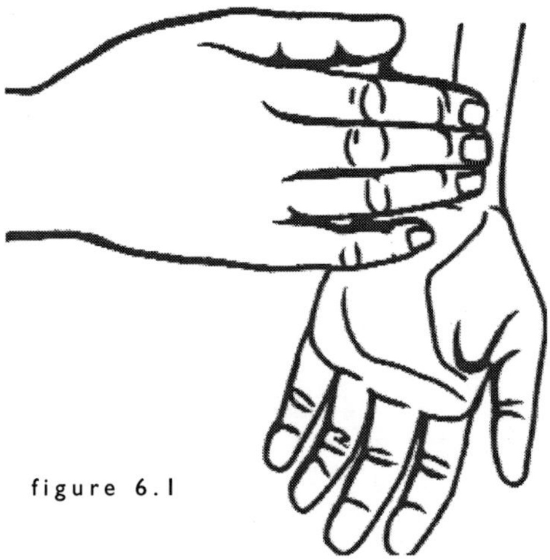

figure 6.1

Taking a pulse:

- Use the first three fingers of one hand, and hold them against the patient's radial artery which is located on the thumb side of her inner wrist
- Ask the patient to hold her arm still while you locate her pulse, which will feel like a gentle throb
- Using a watch or clock with a second hand, count the number of beats for 60 seconds
- Report abnormal pulse rates to the patient's doctor

Respiration

Respiration is the process of breathing air into and out of the lungs. The number of times the patient inhales and exhales can be significant in determining whether a problem exists. In an adult, normal respiration is 12 to 20 breaths per minute. Respirations should be quiet and effortless.

Factors affecting respiration:

- presence of heart or respiratory disease
- emotional stress
- heat and cold
- exercise
- infection, fever, or illness

Breathing difficulties are very uncomfortable and distressing to the patient. The feeling of not being able to get an adequate amount of oxygen when inhaling (breathing in) creates a fear that can quickly lead to a state of anxiety or panic. Anxiety will make breathing even more difficult. There are measures that can lessen some of the patient's discomfort and anxiety associated with breathing difficulties.

Measures that help alleviate breathing difficulties:

- Provide a relaxed environment. Speak softly and calmly.
- Keep the home as dust free and clean as possible.
- Allow for adequate ventilation; e.g., open windows or turn on a fan.
- Use an air conditioner in hot or humid weather.
- Administer prescribed inhalers, nebulizers, or other medications.
- Loosen the patient's clothing. Remove unnecessary layers of clothing.
- Keep the thermostat at a setting comfortable to the patient.
- A humidifier or bowl of water placed in the patient's room will keep the air from becoming too dry.
- Sitting upright in a chair or bed allows the lungs to expand more completely and will make breathing easier.

Counting Respirations:

1. Using a watch or clock with a second hand, begin counting the patient's respirations.
2. Each time the patient's chest rises (inhalation) and falls (exhalation) counts as one respiration.
3. If the patient's respirations are shallow or difficult to see, place your hand on her chest and feel it rise and fall.
4. Continue counting the respirations for a full minute. Normal respiration for an adult is 12 to 20 breaths per minute.

☞ *Remember:*

IF THE PATIENT IS EXPERIENCING BREATHING DIFFICULTIES, NOTIFY A DOCTOR.

Giving Medication

Medications are divided into two categories: prescription and nonprescription. Prescription drugs are given to the patient only under the orders and supervision of a doctor. Nonprescription drugs can be purchased "over the counter (OTC)."

We recommend that you check with the patient's doctor before giving her *any* OTC medications, as certain prescription and nonprescription drugs when taken in combination can produce serious side effects.

Your job as the caregiver is to make sure the patient's medications are taken correctly. Certain guidelines must be followed to ensure that medication errors are not made.

- Know why the patient is taking the medication.
- Know the possible side effects of the medication the patient is taking.
- Always read the medication label and any leaflets or information accompanying it.
- Ensure that you have the correct medication.
- Ensure that the exact amount of prescribed medication is given.
- Adhere to the recommended times that the medication is to be given.
- Check the expiration date. Do not use the medication if it has expired.
- Follow storage instructions. Some medications must be stored in the refrigerator. Keep all medications out of direct sunlight and areas of excessive moisture or heat.
- Dispose of medications not used, or those that the doctor has discontinued.
- Keep each medication in its separate, labeled, child-proof container.

- Do not crush pills or open capsules unless the patient's doctor or pharmacist has approved this.
- Call the doctor's office or pharmacist if you have any questions or concerns regarding the patient's medication.

Administering medications can be confusing, especially if there are several different medications that must be given at different times. Forgetting to give the patient her medication or giving extra doses can be very dangerous. Pre-filling a medication dispenser (pill box) or preparing a medication schedule can eliminate confusion and avoid errors.

Medication Dispensers

Medication dispensers are plastic boxes that can be pre-filled with the patient's pills on a daily or weekly basis. Medication dispensers are relatively inexpensive and can be purchased at drug stores or variety stores.

Medication Schedule

A medication schedule is an easy-to-use form that allows you to keep accurate records of the medication the patient is taking, and the times the medication should be given. The medication schedule on page 77 can be photocopied and used to set up your patient's schedule.*

*Visit www.epill.com/schedule.html to download a free medication planner. Additional medication monitoring devices are available to purchase at this web site.

Medication Schedule - fill in the name of the drug and the amount to be taken:

	Sunday	Monday	Tuesday	Wednesday	Thursday	Friday	Saturday
Morning							
Afternoon							
Evening							
Bedtime							

Guidelines for Giving an Injection (Shot)

1. Wash your hands. Wear disposable gloves
2. Using a circular motion, cleanse the injection site with rubbing alcohol and a cotton ball, or prepackaged alcohol wipes
3. Alternate the site of injection to ensure proper absorption of the medication. Giving the injection in the same area repeatedly will cause scar tissue to develop below the skin's surface, thus affecting the proper absorption of the medication
4. If you use the patient's abdomen as an injection site, do not give the shot within one inch of the umbilicus (belly button)
5. Use a new needle and syringe for each injection
6. Do not try to recap the needle following an injection. This practice significantly increases the risk of a needle stick
7. Dispose of used needles immediately. Put used needles in a container that is hard, plastic, and puncture-resistant. Special biohazard containers can be obtained from a hospital, clinical laboratory, drug store, or medical supply store. Check with your local waste disposal program for any special instructions for discarding the container
8. Call the patient's doctor if you have any questions or concerns about giving an injection

Heat and Cold Applications

Heat and cold applications are simple and effective comfort measures that can relieve pain, or can be used to treat injured body tissue. They should be used only with a doctor's approval.

Heat and cold applications are either dry or moist, and can be applied in various forms. The patient's doctor will instruct you on the proper type of therapy.

Tell the patient to report immediately any discomfort while heat or cold is being applied. Check the involved skin every 5 minutes. Remove the heat or cold if the patient's skin becomes red, pale, bluish, or if the patient complains of pain or numbness.

Heat Therapy

Heat increases blood flow and helps bring nutrients and oxygen to the area where heat is being applied. Heat produces its maximum benefits in 20 to 30 minutes. Lengthening the time or increasing the temperature can cause serious damage to the patient's skin.

☞ *Remember:*

DO NOT APPLY HEAT TO THE SKIN COVERING METAL IMPLANTS, SUCH AS PACEMAKERS OR JOINT REPLACEMENTS. DEEP BURNS CAN OCCUR.

Types of Heat Applications

Warm tub bath or shower: Warm baths and showers are a simple and convenient way to relieve pain and relax the body. This method works well for the patient with a sprain, muscle aches or spasms, or hemorrhoids. A bath or shower also helps to relieve back pain and joint stiffness.

☞ *Remember:*

WARM TUB BATHS OR SHOWERS CAN CAUSE THE PATIENT TO FEEL LIGHT-HEADED OR WEAK. ENSURE THE PATIENT'S SAFETY AT ALL TIMES.

Warm, moist compresses: Warm moist compresses consist of a washcloth or small towel that is thoroughly dampened with warm water. Moist compresses can be used for eye irritation or to reduce swelling.

Heating pads: Heating pads can be used for the patient with low back pain or muscle aches. They are lightweight and conform to body contours. Newer heating pads on the market will automatically shut off after twenty minutes.

- Keep the pad at a low to medium setting.
- Do not fold the pad. This can cause the heating unit to malfunction.
- Always make sure the heating pad is covered with a flannel or cotton case. A heating pad should never be in direct contact with the patient's skin.
- Do not use safety pins to attach the heating pad to clothing, bedding, or upholstery.
- Do not use a heating pad near water because of the possibility of electrocution.
- Never allow the patient to sit or lie on a heating pad. Heat will accumulate and may cause burns.

Hot Water Bottles: Hot water bottles can be used for the patient with deep muscle or ligament pain.

- Fill the hot water bottle two thirds full with water heated to a comfortable temperature.
- Cover the bottle with a towel.
- Lean the hot water bottle against the painful area instead of laying it on top of the area.

Cold Therapy

Cold therapy decreases blood flow and allows for deep muscle penetration. Do not allow cold applications to remain on the patient's skin longer than her doctor has specified.

☞ *Remember:*

COLD RUNNING WATER, APPLIED IMMEDIATELY, CAN DECREASE TISSUE DAMAGE FROM MINOR BURNS.

Types of Cold Applications

Cold, moist compresses: Cold moist compresses can be used to relieve pain and swelling in joints, reduce fever, and decrease the discomforts of itchy skin.

To prepare and apply a cold compress:

1. Wash your hands
2. Soak a washcloth or towel in cold water
3. Squeeze the excess water out, and apply the compress to the affected area
4. Rewet the compress frequently, as it will warm from the patient's body heat

☞ *Remember:*

STOP TREATMENT IF YOU NOTICE UNUSUALLY RED, PALE, BLUISH SKIN, OR IF THE PATIENT COMPLAINS OF DISCOMFORT OR INCREASED PAIN.

Cold packs: Cold packs can be used for sprains, muscle spasms, arthritis, and after bone and joint surgery. A washcloth, towel, or pillow case should be placed between the cold pack and the patient's skin to provide comfort, absorb moisture from the outside of the pack, and to protect the skin. Commercial cold packs can be purchased at variety stores or medical supply stores.

To make your own cold pack:

- Fill a plastic bag with ice cubes. Seal the bag
- A frozen bag of peas makes an excellent cold pack because it easily molds to any curved body part
- Moisten 4-inch square gauze pads with water. Freeze them in a plastic bag. Use them to apply cold to a finger, nose, knee, or ankle

Remember:

COLD-INDUCED NUMBNESS MAY MAKE THE PATIENT FEEL LIKE INCREASING ACTIVITY TO THE INJURED AREA. CAUTION THE PATIENT AGAINST THIS PRACTICE UNTIL HEALING HAS OCCURRED.

Summary

In summary, monitoring the patient's temperature, pulse, and respiration can alert you to a problem in its early stages. Errors in giving medication can be avoided if you are conscientious and adhere to simple safety measures. Heat and cold applications, used with a doctor's approval, can relieve pain and help treat injured body tissue.

Chapter 7

Comfort Measures

The comfort needs of the patient must be considered a priority.

In this chapter, you will learn

- how to prevent pressure sores and keep the skin healthy
- how correct body alignment promotes healthy circulation, comfort, and reduces pressure
- why controlling pain is necessary to improve or maintain the patient's quality of life

Prevention of Pressure Sores/Skin Care

Pressure sores will occur if the patient remains in the same position for too long. Pressure sores are the result of an insufficient amount of nutrients and blood flow to a particular area of the body.

Additional causes of pressure sores:

- rubbing or friction from repositioning
- very dry or moist skin
- skin irritation from urine or feces

Common sites of pressure sores:

- over bony areas, such as the back of the head, the shoulders, elbows, lower back, tailbone, buttocks, hips, ankles, heels, and toes
- between abdominal folds, under the breasts

Patients at risk:

- elderly or immobile
- obese or very thin
- malnourished, depressed, or confused
- patients in casts, braces, or splints
- patients with decreased ability to feel pain or pressure; e.g., stroke or diabetic patients

Early signs of pressure sores:

- a pale, red, inflamed, or darkened area
- the involved area is warm to the touch
- a blister or crack is present
- the patient complains of tenderness, burning, or tingling

Preventing pressure sores:

- Reposition the patient every 2 hours.
- Keep the patient's skin clean and dry.
- Apply lotion to the patient's skin to promote circulation and avoid excessive dryness.
- Keep the patient's bedding free of wrinkles and objects that could cause skin irritation.
- Ensure that braces, splints, and shoes fit properly.
- Encourage good nutrition and adequate fluid intake.

Treating a Pressure Sore

Once a pressure sore has developed, the patient's doctor should decide the course of treatment. Caring for a pressure sore will vary from medications and whirlpools to dressing changes and surgical procedures.

☞ Remember:

A PRESSURE SORE IS DIFFICULT TO HEAL. THE BEST TREATMENT IS PREVENTION.

Correct Body Alignment/Positioning

If the patient is elderly, ill, injured, or immobile, you will need to assist him to be properly positioned in his bed or wheelchair, and to maintain correct body alignment. Proper positioning will increase the patient's comfort and circulation, and reduce pressure on various areas of the body.

Positioning the patient in a wheelchair:

1. Place a cushion or small pillow in the wheelchair seat.
2. Position the patient's hips to the back of the wheelchair, with his feet resting on the foot rests or floor.
3. Place a small pillow on one or both sides of the patient, to prevent him from leaning sideways.
4. The patient's arms should be placed on the wheelchair arm rests, or on a pillow placed across his lap.

Positioning the patient in bed:

Semi-sitting (head of the bed elevated 45-60 degrees)

1. The patient's back should be straight, with a small pillow placed under his head.
2. Place two pillows, one on each side of the patient, for his arms to rest on.
3. Place a pillow under the patient's calves so that his heels aren't resting on the bed.

Back-lying

1. The patient's legs should be straight and in alignment with his head and back.
2. Place a pillow under the patient's head, neck, and upper shoulders.
3. Place two pillows, one on each side of the patient, for his arms to rest on.
4. A pillow may be placed under the patient's knees for additional comfort.
5. Place a pillow under the patient's calves so that his heels aren't resting on the bed.

Side-lying

1. Place a pillow under the patient's head and neck.
2. The patient's upper leg should be bent at his knee, and a pillow placed beneath it.
3. The patient's upper arm should be bent at the elbow, and a pillow placed beneath it.
4. A pillow should be placed behind the patient's back to prevent him from rolling back.
5. Ensure that the patient's lower arm and leg are in a comfortable position.

In addition to using pillows to maintain good body alignment, there are other comfort devices that can be used:

- Heel and elbow protectors cushion the heels and elbows from the hard surface of the bed.
- Air mattresses help to distribute the patient's body weight evenly, thus preventing pressure to any one area.

Remember:

IF THE PATIENT LOOKS UNCOMFORTABLE, HE PROBABLY IS.

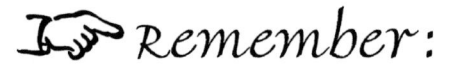

Pain Control

Often the patient's greatest fear is the prospect of coping with pain. Knowing that medication is available to help minimize his pain is reassuring to the patient. Remember that pain is a symptom that only the patient can identify and describe. If the patient complains of pain, notify his doctor.

It is difficult to assess pain in a confused or nonverbal patient. Look for other cues, such as wrinkling of the eyebrow, facial grimacing, increased fatigue, irritability, sleep disturbances, or depression. Culture, religion, and the patient's support system may also influence his response to pain. Be understanding of the patient's need to express pain in his own way.

☞ *Remember:*

IF THE PATIENT DOES NOT SHOW OBVIOUS SIGNS OF PAIN, IT DOES NOT MEAN THAT HE IS WITHOUT PAIN.

Facts about Pain

- Pain is the body's way of showing that all is not well.
- Chronic pain, left untreated, can cause the patient to become depressed, angry, frustrated, dependent, and withdrawn.
- Anxiety increases pain, and pain increases anxiety.

Pain Medication

The doctor will prescribe a pain medication that will be most appropriate for the patient's needs. Give the pain medication to the patient as the doctor prescribes it. Pain medicine is not as effective if you wait until the patient's pain is severe before giving the medicine.

When to call the doctor:

- if the patient's pain increases or the medication is not providing relief
- if you notice side effects from the pain medication the patient is taking
- if the patient appears overmedicated; e.g., he exhibits increased confusion or excessive drowsiness

Summary

In summary, making the patient more comfortable will improve his quality of life. Conscientious skin care will help to prevent skin breakdown. Proper positioning and correct body alignment can prevent painful pressure sores. You can minimize the physical discomforts of pain by administering the patient's pain medication as prescribed by the doctor.

Chapter 8

Communication

Communication is the sharing of information with another person. It can be either verbal (using words) or nonverbal (using body language). Communicating will allow you and the patient to express emotions and make your wishes known to one another.

You may be caring for a patient with impaired senses. Vision difficulties, for example, can disrupt the patient's ability to carry out simple tasks safely. Hearing difficulties often result in the patient having inadequate information about her disease process, leading to noncompliance with instructions that are pertinent to maintaining good health. Speech difficulties limit the patient's ability to express her needs. Impaired thinking affects the patient's ability to problem-solve, remember, and use good judgment. Patients with Alzheimer's disease and other dementias often exhibit negative or uncooperative behavior making communication very challenging.

In this chapter you will learn

- alternate ways to communicate effectively with a patient who has impaired vision, hearing, speech, and/or thought
- how the patient's body language can communicate to you
- ways to decrease difficult and disruptive behavior

Impaired Vision, Hearing and Speech

Impaired vision, hearing, and speech are conditions experienced by many elderly, ill, or injured patients. You can improve communication and help the patient become more independent if you learn how to adjust to her impairments.

Communicating with the Vision-Impaired Patient

1. Stand directly in front of the patient when talking to her.
2. Let the patient know you are present by speaking in a normal tone of voice.
3. Tell the patient beforehand if you will be touching her, as abrupt touch can be startling.
4. Inform the patient when you will be leaving the room.
5. Tell the patient about any changes made in her room or furnishings.
6. Explain all unusual sounds the patient hears, but cannot see.
7. Provide activities that stimulate the patient's other senses, such as listening to music, sampling tasty food, and feeling different fabrics and textures.

Aids for the vision-impaired patient:*

- Prescription lenses should be checked regularly by a professional to see if they are still an appropriate strength.
- Clocks and watches with raised dots allow the patient to "feel" the time of day, and can be purchased at medical supply stores.
- Large print books and audio books are available through most public libraries or book clubs.
- There are many specialized tools available that allow the patient to perform tasks that normally require good vision; e.g., a tool for signing checks or addressing envelopes. They can be ordered through a medical supply company.
- Magnifiers help the patient read small print.

* Internet resources for aids include www.independentliving.com, which sells a variety of aids for grooming, mobility, and reading; and www.lowvision.org/independent-living-aids.htm, which contains links to sites that sell and provide aids for the visually impaired.

Communicating with the Hearing-Impaired Patient

- Let the patient know you are present, by moving near her so that you can be seen, or by gently touching her.
- Before you speak, turn down all background noises, such as radios and television.
- Provide adequate lighting in the room so the patient can see your face and read your lips.
- Speak in a natural manner, and use simple sentences.
- If the patient has some hearing ability in one ear, position yourself on her "good" side.
- Use sign language or facial expressions to communicate.
- Do not cover your mouth, chew gum, or turn away while you are communicating with the patient.
- Provide the patient with paper and pencil or a small chalkboard.

Aids for the hearing-impaired patient:

- Consult the patient's doctor about her need for hearing aids.
- A special telephone with a flashing light indicates that the phone is ringing.
- Amplifiers increase the sound of a television, radio, or telephone. Special telephones and amplifiers can be purchased at electronics stores.**

Communicating with the Speech-Impaired Patient

- Be patient. Give the patient adequate time to finish her sentences. Do not interrupt or speak for her.
- Encourage the patient to participate in conversation, using whatever means she is capable of. This will help her feel worthwhile.
- Pay attention to the patient's nonverbal communication (body language).

** An internet resource for these amplifiers is www.lifewithease.com/fithear.html.

Aids for the speech-impaired patient:

- Keep a pencil and paper, small chalkboard, and a bell within reach of the patient.
- Use flashcards. These can easily be made by taping magazine pictures of frequently used items onto blank index cards; e.g., a glass of orange juice (to indicate thirst) or a picture of a pill (to indicate pain).

☞ Remember:

FREQUENT COMPLIMENTS WILL REINFORCE THE PATIENT'S STRENGTHS AND FEELINGS OF ACCOMPLISHMENT.

Alternate Ways to Communicate (Nonverbal Cues)

Touch: Touch can be a powerful therapy if it is used at the proper time. Touching can communicate warmth and friendliness, openness, empathy, and competence.

Eye contact: Eye contact shows the patient that you are willing to listen. Lack of eye contact from the patient may indicate that she is anxious, has hurt feelings, or that she is unwilling to communicate. Remember that in some cultures, eye contact is avoided out of respect for another person.

Facial expressions: The patient's face can show a multitude of expressions such as anger, sadness, fear, and pain. However, the patient may mask her feelings, making it difficult to determine her needs.

Gestures: Grabbing at the throat indicates choking. Clutching at the body or extreme stillness can indicate pain. Turning away can indicate anger or sadness. Wringing the hands or tapping the foot can indicate anxiety.

Remember:

FATIGUE, STRESS, MEDICATION, DISEASE, ILLNESS, AND LANGUAGE BARRIERS CAN AFFECT THE PATIENT'S ABILITY TO EXPRESS HER NEEDS. LOOK FOR NONVERBAL CUES TO HELP YOU DISCOVER THOSE NEEDS.

insight

Nonverbal communication speaks louder than words.

The Confused Patient

The degree of confusion (disorientation) in the patient can range from occasional or temporary forgetfulness to a progressive dementia that inhibits the patient's ability to perform the simplest tasks independently. Communicating with a patient who has an alteration in thought is very challenging. You, as the caregiver, will need to compensate for the patient's diminished ability to communicate.

Tips on communicating with a confused patient:

- Be alert to nonverbal signs of pain or distress, such as frowning, facial grimacing, or moaning.
- Use simple words, pictures and symbols to help the patient understand information; e.g., tape a picture of a toilet to the bathroom door and write the word "bathroom" underneath it.

- Speak quietly and slowly, maintaining eye contact. Give one short, simple instruction to the patient at a time.
- Use only positive words and gestures.
- Do not argue with the patient.
- Give consistent responses.
- Give frequent reminders of the time, day, month, and year using calendars, watches, television, and bulletin boards.
- Use touch when it is appropriate and accepted; e.g., walking arm in arm.
- Keep family pictures or other familiar items in the patient's view to provide security, encourage communication, and to help the patient maintain her identity.
- Allow the patient adequate time to complete sentences and thoughts.
- Avoid reasoning with the patient if it causes her to become upset or anxious.

Strategies to Reduce Difficult Behaviors

Difficult behaviors produce significant stress for caregivers. Managing difficult and disruptive behavior can be one of the greatest challenges in providing care.

What You Can Do:

- Distract the patient by drawing her attention to any familiar object, such as a photograph or favorite piece of furniture.
- Avoid loud television programs, bright lights and continuous chatter as these are disturbing to the patient.
- Use touch as a beneficial therapy to reduce the patient's sense of isolation and anxiety.
- Follow established routines, but allow for flexibility during times when the patient is anxious or agitated.
- Provide simple tasks or activities such as folding towels or frosting cookies.

- Offer the patient a favorite drink or snack. Avoid caffeine.
- Promote bladder and bowel elimination. A full bladder or constipation can increase restlessness and anxiety.
- Do not force the patient into a tub or shower when she is restless or agitated. Bathe her when she is calm.
- Allow meaningful safe wandering to provide exercise. Divert the wandering with adequate rest periods or naps.
- Give the patient opportunities to make choices. Even simple choices will give the patient some control over her life.

☞ Remember:

THE PATIENT MAY NOT BE IN CONTROL OF HER BEHAVIOR OR METHODS OF COMMUNICATION. YOUR REASSURING APPROACH AND KIND WORDS WILL MAKE A DIFFERENCE IN THE WAY SHE RESPONDS TO YOU.

Summary

In summary, impaired vision, hearing, speech, and thought affect the patient's ability to communicate. Despite these impairments, you and the patient can communicate effectively, whether in words or gestures. As with all patients with special needs, the doctor may suggest a specialist who can help the patient improve her abilities to communicate.

☞ Remember:

CALL THE DOCTOR IF YOU NOTICE A SIGNIFICANT CHANGE IN THE PATIENT'S ABILITY TO SEE, HEAR, TALK, OR UNDERSTAND.

Chapter 9

Sleep Disturbances

Inadequate sleep interferes with the patient's ability to restore energy, recover from an illness or surgery, and cope with the demands of the day. There are many factors that affect the patient's ability to get an adequate amount of sleep at night.

In this chapter you will learn

- how to promote effective sleep, so that the patient may function at an optimal level during the day

Factors Affecting Sleep

While there are any number of factors that can affect a patient's ability to sleep at night, here are a few of the most common:

- illness, pain, or discomfort
- psychological problems, such as depression and anxiety
- age (older persons take longer to fall asleep, and awaken more frequently at night)
- dementia, such as Alzheimer's disease
- presence of hunger or thirst
- climate and room temperature
- amount of sleep obtained during the day
- intake of caffeine (tea, cola, coffee), alcohol, or nicotine
- activity and exercise
- excessive stimulation from noise or lighting
- lifestyle and attitude

Signs of Inadequate Sleep

If the patient is able to communicate with you, he may express concerns about not being able to sleep through the night. If he isn't able to communicate with you, or you think he is reluctant to do so, here are some things to watch for:

- poor concentration and memory
- decreased mobility, poor posture
- increased irritability or restlessness
- increased drowsiness, frequent yawning
- dark circles under the eyes
- lack of facial expression
- complaints of difficulty falling asleep, and not feeling rested

☞ Remember:

A SUDDEN CHANGE IN THE PATIENT'S SLEEP PATTERN SHOULD BE REPORTED TO HIS DOCTOR.

Suggestions to Promote Sleep

- Maintain a bedtime routine.
- Encourage the patient to exercise in the afternoon or early evening.
- Avoid beverages containing caffeine, such as coffee, tea, and colas, for 3 to 4 hours before bedtime.
- Offer warm milk or other bedtime snack. Place a glass of water on the bedside table.
- Ensure that the bed sheets and pillow cases are clean, dry, and comfortable, and that the bedding is not too heavy or too light.
- Ensure that the patient is adequately clothed.

- Keep the thermostat at a comfortable temperature (not too warm), and the room adequately ventilated.
- Minimize noise and household activity.
- Do not allow the patient to become overly tired during the day. Encourage and allow short daytime naps, if needed.
- Make sure the patient has taken all his prescribed medication and that pain-relieving medication is within reach (if appropriate for the patient).
- Allow the patient time to talk about any anxiety he is feeling before bedtime.
- Play soft music, offer a book, or read a bedtime story.

☞ Remember:

SLEEPING PILLS SHOULD NOT BE GIVEN TO THE PATIENT WITHOUT THE DOCTOR'S APPROVAL.

Summary

In summary, sleep disturbances prevent the patient from receiving adequate rest, which is vital for his overall well-being. Physical and psychological discomfort, and environmental disturbances, can be minimized if you, the caregiver, are familiar with the most effective ways to promote sleep.

insight

Be good to yourself every day. The rest will come easily.

Chapter 10

Feelings, Emotions, & Social Interactions

Identifying the patient's social support system will allow you to incorporate the love and concern of family and friends into her life. Family and friends are the foundation for improving the patient's self-esteem and her coping abilities. The patient needs to feel secure and productive.

In this chapter, you will learn

- why the patient's sexuality and intimacy concerns are important
- how feelings of depression, anxiety, and guilt can be natural responses to change
- how to help the patient through the grieving process as she copes with loss
- activities to help the patient keep an active mind and spirit

Family and Friends

Family and friends will most likely be the center of the patient's life. Relationships with family and friends that are based on affection and openness will have a positive impact on the patient's well-being. The absence or loss of this support system can lead to extreme loneliness. It is important that every effort be made to allow the patient to have contact with the people most important in her life.

The best way to protect your own health is to achieve balance between meeting your own needs and being a good caregiver. The family and friends of the patient may come to you as the caregiver to offer their help. Often, they are anxious and willing to offer their services, but do not know exactly what is needed, or what they can do. (See Chapter 11 for ways to ask for help.)

What Family and Friends Can Do

- Help with errands, such as grocery shopping or picking up a prescription
- Help with household chores, such as laundry, vacuuming, or doing dishes
- Help with yard work or gardening
- Make a meal or special dessert
- Care for the patient for a short time, so that you can rest or go out
- Visit the patient to boost her morale

Guilt, Depression, and Anxiety

Circumstances may impose some upsetting, but necessary, changes in the patient's life. The patient will respond to change in her own way. Guilt, depression, and anxiety are some of the responses to change the patient may exhibit.

Guilt

Guilt is a feeling of having done something wrong.

Factors that can cause guilt:

- inability to perform personal cares
- inability to provide emotional support to a loved one

- inability to maintain a sexual relationship
- inability to fulfill social commitments
- loss of job or income
- inability to do usual household tasks

Depression

Depression is a feeling of low spirit and hopelessness.

Factors that can cause depression:

- loss of independence
- prolonged illness or permanent injury
- chronic pain
- lack of support from family and friends
- loss of a family member, friend, or pet

Signs of depression:

- loss of interest in pleasure or usual activities
- weight loss or gain
- sleep disturbances or increased fatigue
- stated feelings of worthlessness and guilt
- difficulty concentrating or making decisions
- suicidal comments

☞ Remember:

SUICIDAL COMMENTS MADE BY THE PATIENT SHOULD BE TAKEN SERIOUSLY AND REPORTED TO HER DOCTOR.

Anxiety

Anxiety is a feeling of apprehension or uneasiness. See page 112 for suggestions on relaxation techniques/alternative therapies that are beneficial in decreasing anxiety, restlessness, and feelings of depression.

Factors that can cause anxiety:

- illness, injury, or hospitalization
- change in health status or threat of death
- lack of knowledge and understanding of one's illness
- fear of separation or loss of family or friends

Signs of increased anxiety:

- increased heart rate and breathing rate
- sleep disturbances (See Chapter 9 for information)
- nausea, vomiting, and diarrhea
- frequent urination
- excessive sweating
- trembling, pacing
- angry outbursts or crying

The patient will cope with feelings of guilt, depression, and anxiety based on her individual circumstances of life, personal strengths, and available support system. As the caregiver, you can help by being understanding, supportive, and by encouraging the patient to talk openly about her feelings.

Grief

Grieving is a natural, healthy, emotional response to loss. At any stage of life loss may occur. As the patient ages, the amount of time it takes to recover from loss increases. Loss of independence, a body part, finances, social status, job productivity, a spouse or other family member, are examples of loss that will cause the patient to grieve. You as the caregiver are the key person in providing support during the patient's difficult times.

It is important to remember that each patient will cope with loss differently. Many factors —such as culture, faith, religious beliefs, and past methods of coping—influence the way the patient will grieve.

Stages of Grief

1. **Denial:** The patient may respond by acting in disbelief. E.g., "The doctor must have made a mistake." She may experience a feeling of emotional "numbness" or shock.
2. **Anger:** The patient may respond with feelings of resentment. She may be angry at herself for not preventing the loss, or she may direct her anger toward you.
3. **Bargaining:** The patient may respond by trying to negotiate away the loss by making promises to God or fate. E.g., "I'll never smoke another cigarette if you'll let me make it to my son's wedding." She may also have feelings of guilt or self-blame.
4. **Depression:** The patient may respond by crying or withdrawing from usual activities. She may feel physically and mentally exhausted. Keep in mind that despite your efforts to comfort and support the patient, she may benefit from talking to a health care professional, counselor, or someone who has suffered similar losses. Know your limitations and abilities. Don't be afraid to ask for help.
5. **Acceptance:** The patient may respond by preparing a will, allowing visitors, or showing more interest in her personal cares. She will continue to feel the loss, but it will be easier for her to cope with it.

insight

Touch, offered freely, will convey both compassion and reassurance.

Helping the patient cope with grief:

- Encourage the patient to express her feelings.
- Encourage independence. Involve the patient in decision making.
- Arrange for visits with the patient's minister, priest, or spiritual advisor.
- Be a good listener. Do not be judgmental.
- Help the patient to focus on her strengths and set realistic goals.
- Acknowledge the patient's fears and concerns.
- Keep familiar and special objects in the patient's view to help her feel more secure.
- Encourage exercise, good eating habits, and adequate rest.
- Be patient and offer reassurance.

Self-Esteem

Self-esteem is the way a person feels about herself.

Factors that decrease self-esteem:

- illness, injury, or disability
- inadequate love and support
- loss of independence and control
- age-related body changes
- unrealistic expectations
- any form of abuse

To improve the patient's self-esteem:

- Show genuine concern for the patient's feelings.
- Give sincere compliments.
- Allow the patient to make decisions and choices.
- Spend uninterrupted time with the patient (unrelated to providing personal cares).
- Arrange for social interactions with family and friends.

Intimacy and Sexuality

Age, illness, and injury do not diminish the patient's need for feelings of love and belonging. Sexual needs and desires are a natural and normal part of the patient's life.

Intimacy for the patient and her partner includes the sharing of warm and caring feelings, whether they be physical or emotional. Feeling important and wanted by another person will give the patient a sense of comfort and security. Healthy sexuality and intimacy depends on freedom from guilt and anxiety. If the patient has questions or concerns about issues related to sexuality and intimacy, call the patient's doctor, a counselor, or sex therapist.

Misconceptions about Sexuality

- Older people do not desire or enjoy sex.
- Older people do not need to feel attractive or sexually appealing.
- Injured or disabled people are not capable of having sex.

Remember:

SOME MEDICATIONS HAVE SIDE EFFECTS THAT MAY AFFECT THE PATIENT'S SEXUAL ABILITY AND DESIRE.

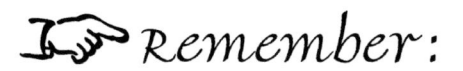

Spiritual Needs

Spiritual and religious beliefs affect the patient's behavior in health and illness. As the caregiver, it is important that you accept the patient's values and support her religious practices. The patient's religious faith can be vital in helping her to accept and cope with her condition.

To meet the patient's spiritual needs:

- Respect the patient's need for privacy during prayer.
- Arrange for visits from clergy.
- Support any religious practice that is meaningful to the patient, as long as it does not cause harm.
- Obtain reading material or cassettes tapes of sermons and hymns from her religious institution.
- Arrange for the patient to receive the sacraments, if that is her wish.
- Keep objects at the bedside that provide spiritual comfort, such as a Bible, rosary beads, statues, or pictures.

Entertainment

Regardless of the patient's health or age, social interactions should take place. Consider the patient's cultural, social, and ethnic background when planning entertainment.

Suggestions for Entertainment

There are a variety of activities that can occupy the patient's time and fulfill her need to be active. Suggestions for activities the patient may be able to engage in independently are:

- listening to audio books (can be rented from the local library)
- folding/sorting laundry

- washing/drying dishes
- watering plants
- raking leaves
- organizing dresser/closet/kitchen drawers
- meal preparation
- cutting out cookies
- knitting, crocheting, embroidery
- solitaire and other card games
- browsing through mail order catalogs
- watching TV or movies on dvd
- writing notes to friends or sending e-mails
- listening to music
- setting the table
- woodworking, stenciling or other craft projects

Suggestions for activities you can engage in with the patient include:

- Make a scrapbook with the patient, or look at pictures from the past.
- Invite friends or family members to eat lunch with the patient.
- Call friends or family of the patient, so that she may talk to them.
- Help the patient write letters to distant friends or family.
- Join a support group or organization with the patient.
- Take the patient to a park to watch the children play.
- Share an ice cream treat with the neighbors.
- Cut and arrange fresh flowers in a vase for the patient's room.
- Draw or color a picture together.
- Play cards, bingo, work puzzles, play board games, or do crafts.
- Research topics on the Internet.
- Have sing-a-longs.

- Exercise to lively music.
- Plant a garden.

☞ Remember:

THE SUPPORT AND ATTITUDES OF FAMILY AND FRIENDS HAVE AN IMPACT ON THE PATIENT'S COURSE OF ILLNESS AND RECOVERY PERIOD.

Summary

In summary, the patient's age, illness, or the presence of injury may require family members to assume new roles and responsibilities. The need for increased care, and the decreased ability of the patient to engage in social activities, can result in decreased self-esteem, and feelings of depression, anxiety, and guilt. Recognizing and understanding the stages of grief will enable you to support the patient as she goes through the grieving process.

in**sight**

A loving family and loyal friends are irreplaceable treasures.

Chapter 11

Taking Care of the Caregiver

Accepting the role as caregiver may be one of the most challenging jobs you will ever undertake. Rarely will your caregiving role become routine. Many demands will confront you on a daily basis. In this chapter, you will learn

- how you can maintain a healthy mind and body
- how to understand your needs and recognize your limitations
- how to identify the signs of role strain and how to deal with it

Healthy Mind and Body

Health and wellness mean more than not being ill. They mean achieving the maximum potential of your physical, mental, emotional, and spiritual well being. While your role as a caregiver will enhance the quality of life for the patient, you should not neglect your own health. Your mind and body will function at their best if you strive to meet your basic human needs. Satisfying these needs will give you the strength and ability to cope with your very challenging and difficult role.

Physical Needs

Physical needs include breathing, the intake and output of food and fluids, and sleep.

To help meet your physical needs:

- Eat three nutritious meals each day.
- Drink eight, 8-ounce glasses of fluid every day.
- Get adequate sleep and rest.
- Have a quiet time to relax every day.
- Spend time outdoors, weather permitting.
- Exercise every day, preferably away from the patient. Try yoga, or just walk around the block.
- Have regular medical and dental checkups.

Emotional Needs

Emotional needs involve the expression of your feelings, such as love, belonging, happiness, sadness, loneliness, and fear. Stress and anxiety will put a strain on your body and affect your health. Relaxation, calm behavior, and laughter will strengthen your body's response to illness and help you to cope effectively.

To help meet your emotional needs:

- Share your feelings and needs with others.
- Don't be afraid to cry.
- Ask for, and accept help from others.
- Take time for yourself every day.
- Maintain contact with your friends and family.
- Consider joining a support group or organization.

☞ Remember:

IT IS IMPORTANT THAT YOU FIND SOMEONE WHO WILL LISTEN TO YOU AND ALLOW YOU TO TALK ABOUT YOUR FEELINGS.

Intellectual Needs

Intellectual needs include thinking, making decisions, learning, and solving problems.

To help meet your intellectual needs:

- Read magazines or books, work crossword puzzles, or play cards or board games.
- Renew interest in a past hobby or learn a new one.
- Draw a picture, write a poem, or listen to music.
- Learn how to use a computer.

Environmental Needs

Environmental needs involve your physical surroundings. Housing, neighborhood, climate, temperature, sanitation, and feelings of safety will have an impact on your health. (See Chapter 14, Resource Information.)

To help meet your environmental needs:

- Contact community agencies to get information about energy and heating assistance.
- Many communities offer low income housing.
- Contact community support groups or organizations to get help with home improvements, such as winterization of the home, and the building of wheelchair ramps.

Social/Cultural Needs

Social/cultural needs deal with relationships and communication. Frequent contact with people you trust will provide you with a sense of belonging. Your income level, lifestyle, family, friends, and culture will have an impact on your health practices.

To help meet your social/cultural needs:

- Practice your cultural beliefs and traditions.
- Spend time with your family and friends.
- Arrange time away from your caregiver role to do what you enjoy, such as having your hair done or seeing a movie.

Spiritual Needs

Spiritual needs involve your values and beliefs as they relate to a higher being. Your spirituality can influence the way you respond to health and illness, as well as to taking care of others' needs.

To help meet your spiritual needs:

- Allow yourself adequate time and privacy to practice your faith.
- Talk to or visit your clergy.

Alternative Therapies

There are many complimentary and alternative ways to reduce stress and provide comfort and relaxation. Additional information regarding alternative therapies can be obtained from the library, bookstores, the Internet, local newspaper or yellow pages of the telephone book.

Massage Therapy: Therapeutic massage is relaxing, improves immune function, and can decrease feelings of anxiety and restlessness.

Music Therapy: Listening to soothing music can boost the immune system by reducing stress. Music has been shown to help relieve symptoms of depression and anxiety.

Tai Chi: People of all ages and levels of well-being may practice Tai Chi. The movements involved look similar to a slow, deliberate form of dance. These movements, along with special techniques of breathing and mental focus, help to relax, build stamina, flexibility and balance.

Yoga: Yoga is a therapeutic exercise program that teaches restful poses and breathing techniques. Increased mobility, neck strength and easier breathing are some of the benefits of yoga. The practice of yoga is all about creating union between your body, mind and spirit, thus facilitating health, happiness, and a deeper connection to one's life.

Nia: Neuromuscular Integrative Action is founded on the concept that there is a dancer, martial artist, and highly aware person within you. By melding various concepts together, Nia sets this person free.

insight

Cry today, but laugh tomorrow.

Understanding Your Limits

Caregiving can be physically and emotionally exhausting. It can change every aspect of your life. The patient's condition can decline, causing an increased dependency on you, making your role as caregiver more difficult. Circumstances in your life can change and may interfere with your ability to provide good care.

Realize that your own needs must be met before you can be an effective caregiver. Know your limits. Don't feel guilty or think that you have failed in your obligations if you can no longer care for the patient in the home. Arranging for alternative care may be in the best interests of both the patient and yourself.

Identifying Role Strain

Caregiver role strain is a term used to describe a situation in which you experience difficulties in performing your role as a caregiver. Conflict can occur if your expectations about your role are not clear, if your goals are unrealistic, or if your responsibilities become overwhelming.

Factors leading to caregiver role strain:

- feeling that you don't have a choice
- difficulty doing the work that is expected of you
- lack of help and support
- feeling that your efforts are unsuccessful or unappreciated
- interference with your personal and/or work life
- lack of physical resources, such as youth and strength
- poor relationship between you and the patient
- loss of companionship
- becoming physically and/or emotionally drained

Signs of caregiver role strain:

- difficulty sleeping
- problems concentrating or making decisions
- low tolerance level; easily frustrated
- fatigue or loss of energy
- drug or alcohol use
- weight loss or gain
- loss of pride and interest in providing care
- feelings of loneliness and isolation

☞ Remember:

CAREGIVER ROLE STRAIN CAN LEAD TO PATIENT NEGLECT OR MISTREATMENT. A DOCTOR OR COUNSELOR CAN OFFER HELP IF YOU ARE EXPERIENCING THE SIGNS OF CAREGIVER ROLE STRAIN.

Role Reversal

Roles within a relationship can change suddenly or gradually because of an illness or disability. When a parent you have always looked to for strength and guidance becomes frail or sick, it is difficult and frightening to accept the responsibility of caring for him or her. When the spouse you have always relied upon as provider and protector can no longer function in that role, you may feel obligated to assume the role of provider and protector.

Role reversals can be difficult to cope with and accept. Don't try to cope with role reversals by yourself. Ask for help from family, friends, and support groups or organizations. See Chapter 14 for more information on support groups or organizations.

Asking for help and utilizing any available resources will strengthen your relationship with the patient, reduce your stress level, and make coping with your job as a caregiver more manageable.

Community/Home Resources

See Chapter 14 for Resource Information on the following services:

In Home Sitting provides companionship and temporary care for the patient. Sitting services usually include both day and nighttime hours.

Adult Day Care centers provide a break (respite) to the caregiver while providing health services, therapeutic services, and social activities for people with Alzheimer's disease and related dementia, chronic illnesses, traumatic brain injuries, developmental disabilities, and other problems that increase their care needs. Some adult day care centers are dementia specific, providing services exclusively to that population.

Housekeeping Services offer help with laundry, vacuuming, and other household duties, as well as grocery shopping and meal preparation.

Meal Service provides a nutritious meal that is either delivered to the patient's home or is served in a group setting, five or more days a week.

Family Medical Leave Act of 1993 allows you up to 12 weeks of unpaid job-protected leave to care for a family member.

Home Health Care is a provider of Home Health Services in the Medicare program. Home Health Care can provide the patient with a registered nurse, home health aide, a physical therapist, occupational therapist, speech therapist, respiratory therapy, and a medical social worker to assist in meeting the patient's needs. Home Health Care costs are usually fully reimbursed by private insurance, Medicare, Medicaid, or other funding source.

Note: Your home health agency will be responsible for providing and arranging for all of your necessary therapy services and medical supplies.

1. Nursing services include:

- Collection of laboratory samples
- Injections
- Catheter and ostomy care

- Blood sugar testing
- Wound care
- Medication administration
- Assistance in administering treatments
- Blood pressure measurements
- IV therapy
- Patient and family education

2. Home Health Aide services include:
- Bathing and dressing
- Hair and nail care
- Exercise assistance

Note: See page 10 for a list of supplies that should be ready prior to a home health aide visit.

3. Physical Therapy services include:
- Assessing the patient's overall mobility level
- Assisting the patient in regaining the best possible joint and muscle function through an individualized program of exercise and activity
- Arranging for supportive devices; e.g., walkers, wheelchairs, and canes

4. Occupational Therapy services include:
- Evaluating the patient's safety needs
- Assisting the patient toward rehabilitation with attention to fine motor skills; e.g., eating and dressing independently
- Arranging for special supportive devices; e.g., eating utensils

5. Speech Therapy services include:
- Assessing swallowing difficulties; e.g., the need for thickened liquids
- Assessing language disabilities; e.g., following a stroke
- Assisting the patient in achieving the optimal ability to communicate

6. Respiratory Therapy services include:
- Monitoring the supply and usage of oxygen
- Monitoring the patient's oxygen levels
- Ensuring the proper functioning of equipment; e.g., exchanging concentrator filters and oxygen tubing

7. Social Worker services include:
- Helping the patient and caregivers adjust and understand the changes and anxieties they may be experiencing
- Assisting in arranging for transportation, meal programs, and other programs of assistance
- Providing information on insurance, financial plans, and other needed arrangements

Hospice offers services such as pain management, spiritual support, counseling, and nursing care. Home sitting or assistance with personal cares may also be available through hospice. Admittance is usually limited to the patient with a terminal illness, such as cancer, lung disease, end-stage heart conditions, and AIDS. Hospice also requires that the patient has a 24-hour caregiver available in the home.

Note: Hospice care has been a fully reimbursable Medicare Part A benefits option for beneficiaries and providers since 1983. Hospice care is also covered by Medicaid in many states.

Assisted Living Facilities are designed for the patient who is able to live on his own, but needs some assistance and supervision. Services may include meal preparation, housekeeping, and laundry. Assisted living facilities are becoming more prevalent, but are not available in every community. Most facilities are private pay or paid through long-term care insurance.

Nursing Homes/Residential Care Homes are facilities that provide complete care for the patient. Some homes are willing to accept patients on a temporary basis. Nursing Homes and Residential Care Homes are sometimes needed for the patient who requires more care and supervision than the in-home caregiver is able to provide.

Summary

In summary, knowing your limitations and taking time for yourself each day will help you to maintain a productive life outside of caregiving. Being able to identify the signs of caregiver role strain can alert you to the need for professional help before a situation becomes a regrettable incident. You can enhance the quality of your life by continually improving your physical, mental, emotional, and spiritual well-being.

Chapter 12

First Aid

Local chapters of the American Red Cross and the American Heart Association offer courses in first aid and cardiopulmonary resuscitation (CPR). In these courses, trained professionals provide you with classroom instruction and allow you hands-on practice of first aid treatments you may need should an emergency situation arise. Having this knowledge will provide you with increased confidence in your role as caregiver. We strongly recommend that you take basic first aid and CPR courses.

In this chapter you will learn

- how to prepare a first aid kit
- how to prepare for an emergency
- basic information on effective first aid treatments for bleeding, choking, burns, a possible broken bone, stroke, seizure, and heart attack

Preparing for an Emergency

- Record all of the patient's medical information, such as her diagnosis, medications she is taking, and any known allergies. Keep this information by the telephone.
- Keep emergency numbers in large print near the telephone, such as 911, Poison Control, Police, and Fire Department. If the telephone is programmable, preprogram emergency numbers and clearly indicate them on the telephone card.
- Have the patient wear a medical I.D. bracelet that alerts emergency personnel to conditions such as diabetes or drug allergies. Your local hospital, pharmacy, or clinic can tell you where to order a bracelet.

- Know the patient's wishes regarding life-sustaining measures, such as CPR or respirators (breathing machines).
- If the patient has an advance directive, such as a Do Not Resuscitate (DNR) order, have a copy available to give to emergency personnel. See Chapter 13 for information on advance directives.

☞ Remember:

CALL 911 IN AN EMERGENCY (IF THIS SERVICE IS AVAILABLE IN YOUR AREA).

Preparing a First Aid Kit

It is reassuring to have a first aid kit readily available before the need for first aid treatment arises. The following first aid supplies should be stored in a clean, plastic container, and kept in a dry place. A first aid kit should be easily accessible to you, but not to a confused patient or to a child. A pharmacist can help you find the needed supplies, or you can purchase a first aid kit that is already prepared. Remember to replace any supplies you use.

First aid supplies:

- 3 rolls of assorted gauze bandages
- 4 individually wrapped non-stick 4x4-inch sterile gauze pads
- assorted adhesive strips
- 3-inch elastic bandage for wrapping a wrist or ankle
- 1 roll each adhesive and paper tape (used for fragile or sensitive skin)
- 1 small box of cotton swabs
- 4 pairs of disposable gloves

- 1 small bottle of hydrogen peroxide (to clean minor wounds)
- antibiotic ointment
- flashlight and batteries (check the batteries periodically)
- scissors, tweezers, safety pins
- a bottle of syrup of ipecac (to induce vomiting if poisons are swallowed); contact the Poison Control Center before giving to the patient
- liquid or powdered activated charcoal (to absorb swallowed poisons); contact the Poison Control Center before giving to the patient

Basic First Aid

Accidents, illness, or injury may require that you respond quickly with a first aid treatment and a phone call for emergency help. You as the caregiver can begin first aid treatments for choking, bleeding, burns, a possible broken bone, stroke, seizure, and heart attack while waiting for emergency help to arrive.

Bleeding

Deep cuts and heavy bleeding are a medical emergency. Your primary goal is to stop the bleeding.

First aid for bleeding:

1. Call for emergency help.
2. Put on disposable gloves.
3. With the palm of your hand, apply firm pressure directly over the wound using a compress, such as a sterile gauze pad or clean hand towel. (See Figure 12.1.)

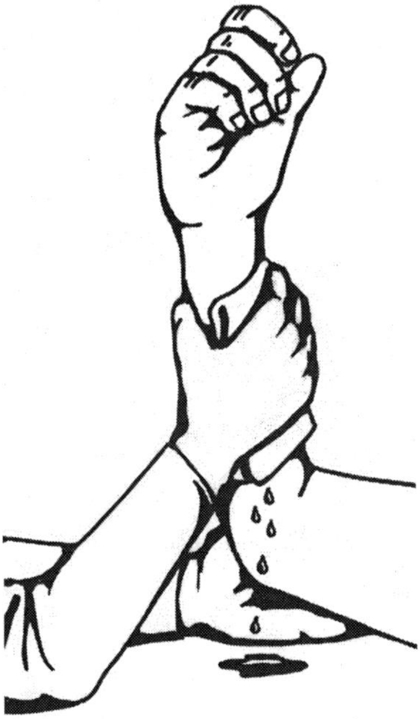

figure 12.1

4. If possible, raise the injured area above the level of the patient's heart. Do not elevate the injured part if you suspect a broken bone.
5. Do not remove the compress if it becomes saturated with blood. Add another compress and apply firmer pressure.
6. Cover and snugly secure the compress by wrapping it with a roll of gauze. Tape the bandage in place.
7. Thoroughly wash your hands after removing the disposable gloves.

☞ Remember:

EVEN MINOR WOUNDS MAY REQUIRE MEDICAL ATTENTION; E.G., TETANUS SHOT, ANTIBIOTICS, OR STITCHES. INFORM THE PATIENT'S DOCTOR OF ALL WOUNDS.

Choking

Choking can be a very frightening experience for both you and the patient. It can quickly become an emergency situation. We will explain the basic steps of the Heimlich Maneuver (abdominal thrusts), the most effective method you can use to dislodge food or other object from the patient's airway. Taking basic CPR and first aid courses will give you additional information and classroom practice of the Heimlich Maneuver (using mannequins).

Signs of choking:

- grabbing at the throat with one or both hands
- inability to talk or difficulty breathing
- wheezing, weak coughing, or high-pitched, squeaky noises
- face becoming red, gray, or blue

First Aid for Choking:

The Heimlich Maneuver is used for adults and for children over one year of age. This procedure should only be done if the patient is unable to breath, talk, or cough. (See Figures 12.2a and 12.2b for the adult procedure.)

1. Call for emergency help.
2. From behind, wrap your arms around the patient's waist.
3. Make a fist and place the thumb side of your fist against the patient's upper abdomen, below the ribcage and above the navel.
4. Grasp your fist with your other hand and press into the upper abdomen with a quick upward thrust. Do not squeeze the ribcage; confine the force of the thrust to your hands.
5. Repeat until object is expelled.

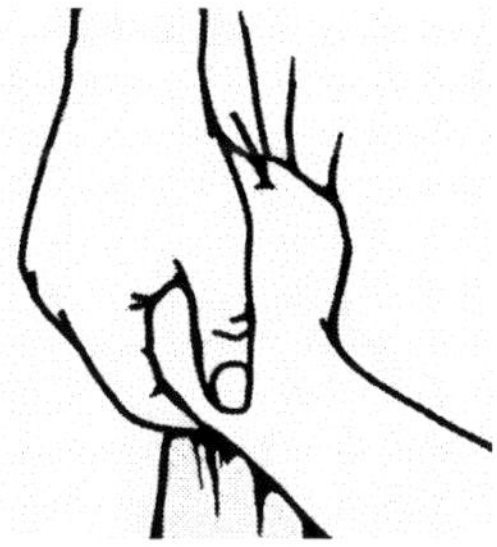

figure 12.2a

figure 12.2B

☞ Remember:

IF THE CHOKING PATIENT IS COUGHING FORCEFULLY, DO NOT INTERFERE. LET HER TRY TO COUGH UP THE OBJECT BY HERSELF.

Burns

Burns are caused by heat, chemicals, electricity, and radiation. Burns are classified under three categories according to their severity.

First Degree Burns: Sun exposure, briefly touching a hot object, and prolonged usage of a hot water bottle or a heating pad can cause a first degree burn. Notify the patient's doctor. Although first degree burns usually heal without treatment, the fragile skin of an elderly patient may need further evaluation.

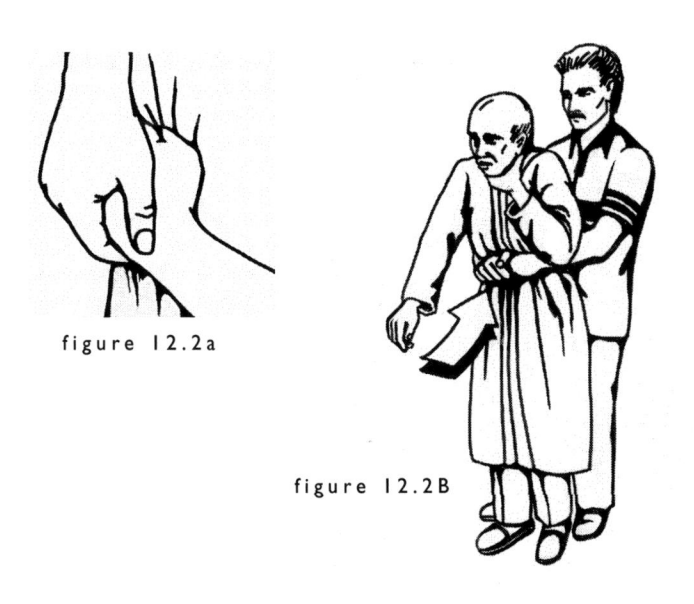

Signs of a first degree burn:

- pink or reddened skin
- pain or discomfort
- mild swelling
- small, thin blisters

☞ Remember:

SUNSCREEN (PROTECTIVE LOTION) SHOULD BE USED TO PREVENT SUNBURN.

Second Degree Burns: Overexposure to the sun, prolonged contact with a hot object, and scalding from steam or hot liquids can cause a second degree burn.

Signs of a second degree burn:

- red, blotchy skin
- large blisters and swelling
- area is moist, shiny, and oozing
- pain

Third Degree Burns: Electrical injury and fire can cause a third degree burn.

Signs of a third degree burn:

- skin may be deep red, white, black, or brown
- skin usually appears dry
- pain varies from extreme to little or none if nerve endings are destroyed

First Aid for Burns: Call 911 or emergency help.

1. Remove the patient from the source of the burn.
2. Cool the burn. Apply large amounts of cool water. Do not use ice or ice water. Apply soaked sheets or other clean cloths to a burned face or other areas that are difficult to immerse in water. Cool the sheets or cloths by adding more water.
3. Cover the burn. Use dry, sterile dressings or clean sheets to cover the burned area.
4. Protect the patient from becoming chilled.

For All Burns:

- Do not apply butter or other home remedies.
- Do not apply pressure.
- Do not remove clothing that is sticking to the burn.
- Do not open blisters or remove dead skin.
- Do not use pain-relieving medications, ointments, or sprays without the doctor's approval.
- Do not cool an electrical burn. Cover the burn with dry, sterile, gauze dressings.

Chemical Burns

Bleach, drain cleaners, lawn, weed, and garden sprays, and paint removers can cause chemical burns.

First Aid for a Chemical Burn:

1. Immediately flush the skin with large amounts of cool, running water (via sink, shower, or garden hose), and call for emergency help.
2. Always flush away from the body. If the patient's eyes are affected, flush from the nose outwards.
3. Remove affected clothing, socks, and shoes.
4. Remove any jewelry that is near the burned area, as swelling may occur.

☞ Remember:

THE LONGER THE CHEMICAL REMAINS ON THE PATIENT'S SKIN, THE WORSE THE BURN WILL BE.

Possible Broken Bone

Seek emergency attention for the patient if you suspect any bone or joint injury. Without x-rays, it is difficult to tell if the injured part is broken.

Signs of a possible broken bone:

- a snapping sound is heard or a snap is felt
- complaints of pain, numbness, or tingling
- inability to move the injured part
- the injured part is abnormally shaped or positioned
- swelling or bruising
- the injured area is cold

☞ Remember:

IF A NECK, BACK, OR HIP INJURY IS SUSPECTED, DO NOT MOVE THE PATIENT. CALL FOR EMERGENCY HELP IMMEDIATELY.

First Aid for a Possible Broken Bone:

1. Do not try to move or straighten the injured part.
2. Support the injured part with pillows or rolled up towels to keep it from moving.
3. Apply ice to the injured area. A towel should be placed between the ice and the patient's skin.
4. Keep the patient warm and comfortable until help arrives.

Stroke

A stroke occurs when there is an interruption of blood flow to the brain. A stroke is a medical emergency. Signs of stroke depend on which area of the brain is involved.

Signs of a stroke:

- severe headache
- drooling, slurred speech, or difficulty swallowing
- weakness, numbness, or loss of the ability to move one or both arms or legs
- loss of bowel or bladder control
- confusion
- visual disturbances
- gradual or sudden loss of consciousness

First Aid for a Stroke:

1. Lay the patient down. Place a pillow under her head and shoulders.
2. Turn the patient onto her side if she is drooling or vomiting.
3. Call for emergency help.
4. Loosen her clothing.
5. Offer comfort and reassurance.
6. Do not give the patient anything to eat or drink.
7. Be prepared to give CPR if the patient loses consciousness and breathing and pulse stop.

Seizures

A seizure occurs when there is a disruption in the normal activity of the brain, causing a loss of body control.

Possible causes of a seizure:

- fever, extreme heat
- injury to the brain
- disease, such as epilepsy or diabetes
- infection

Signs of a seizure:

- aura: an unusual feeling or sensation experienced just before a seizure, such as a visual hallucination or a strange sound or smell
- mild blackout (can be mistaken for daydreaming)
- jerky, involuntary body movements
- uncontrolled muscular contraction

First Aid for a Seizure:

1. Call for emergency help.
2. Protect the patient from injury by removing any nearby objects or safety hazards.
3. Place a folded bath towel under the patient's head.
4. Do not put anything in the patient's mouth or between her teeth.
5. Do not hold or restrain the patient.
6. Place the patient on her side if there is blood, saliva, or vomit in the mouth.
7. Stay with the patient. Provide comfort and reassurance.

Remember:

INCONTINENCE MAY OCCUR WITH A SEIZURE.

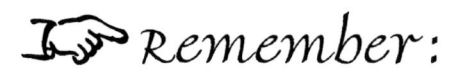

Heart Attack (Myocardial Infarction)

A heart attack occurs when there is an inadequate supply of blood and oxygen to the heart. A heart attack is a medical emergency.

Signs of a heart attack:

- pain or pressure in the chest ranging from discomfort to a crushing, unbearable sensation
- pain that is not relieved with rest or with a change of position
- chest pain that spreads to the neck, jaw, either shoulder or arm, back, or upper abdomen
- shortness of breath
- sweating, pale, or bluish skin
- nausea, vomiting, or complaints of indigestion
- severe anxiety or feeling of impending doom
- extreme weakness or feeling faint

Remember:

NOT EVERYONE WILL SHOW OBVIOUS SIGNS OF A HEART ATTACK. MANY LIVES ARE LOST BECAUSE PEOPLE DENY THEY ARE HAVING A HEART ATTACK, AND WAIT TOO LONG BEFORE SEEKING EMERGENCY HELP.

First Aid for a Heart Attack:

1. Call for emergency help.
2. Place the patient in a semi-sitting or sitting position to make breathing easier. Loosen tight clothing.

3. If the patient's doctor has prescribed nitroglycerin for chest pain, administer the medication as ordered.
4. Be calm and reassure the patient that help is on the way.
5. Do not give the patient anything to eat or drink.
6. If the patient loses consciousness and breathing and pulse stop, be prepared to give CPR.

Remember:

THE TRAINING YOU RECEIVE FROM A CPR COURSE COULD PROVE INVALUABLE IN A HEART ATTACK SITUATION.

Summary

In summary, having an easily accessible first aid kit and knowing how to prepare for an emergency situation will allow you to react more calmly in a stressful situation. Responding quickly with basic first aid for the patient is the most important thing you can do until help arrives.

insight

You cannot do everything, but you can do something.

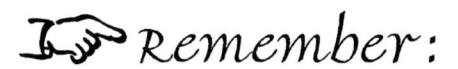

Chapter 13

Legal, Ethical, and Financial Issues

Legal, ethical, and financial decisions about health care can be difficult to make, but with an understanding of the patient's wishes and the options available, these decisions can be made more easily. In this chapter you will learn:

- the patient's rights
- general information related to documents/orders that pertain to medical care decisions
- the financial resources available to the patient

Patient's Rights

1. The patient has all of the rights as a U.S. citizen, such as voting, freedom of religion and speech.
2. The patient has the right to manage his/her own financial affairs.
3. The patient has the right to respect, privacy, and dignity.
4. The patient has the right to be informed of his/her present medical diagnosis, treatment options, and prognosis.
5. The patient has the right to refuse a medical treatment or medication.
6. The patient has the right to be free of physical restraints.
7. The patient has the right to be free of harm and neglect.
8. The patient has the right to participate in social, religious, and community activities.
9. The patient's personal property must be treated with care and respect.

10. The patient has the right to have an Advance Directive.
11. The patient has the right to live in a clean, safe environment.

Advance Directives

Making medical decisions for another person is very difficult. The patient should openly discuss his wishes and feelings regarding life-sustaining measures with close relatives and friends while he is still able. With knowledge about what the patient wants, medical decisions can be made with respect to his choices, which will alleviate confusion and questions about what he "would have wanted."

Advance directives, such as a Living Will and Durable Power of Attorney for Health Care, are legal documents that allow the patient (or a person appointed by the patient) to exercise the right to make medical decisions related to death and the dying process while he is still competent to do so.

The rules for advance directives vary from state to state. The patient's doctor or a lawyer can provide further information and offer guidance as to which advance directive is best for him.*

Living Will

In a living will, the patient directs his doctor to either withhold or withdraw measures that would support or maintain life (other than measures that are necessary for comfort). A living will takes effect if the patient has a critical injury or terminal illness, and death is imminent.

* Information about particular state guidelines for advance directives and additional help with resources and financial planning can be found at the following web site: www.caringinfo.org. At the American Bar Association web site, there is an excellent article by Charles Sabatino, J.D., "10 Legal Myths about Advance Medical Directives." www.abanet.org/aging/myths.html

Durable Power of Attorney for Health Care (DPA)

A written and signed DPA for health care authorizes another individual, such as a spouse, adult child, or other competent person, to make health care decisions on the patient's behalf if he is unable to make decisions independently. It becomes active any time a person is unconscious or unable to make medical decisions. Health care decisions may include the termination of health care and/or life sustaining measures, such as the use of respirators or feeding tubes. A DPA is generally more useful than a living will.

Do Not Resuscitate Orders (DNR)

Do not resuscitate (DNR) means that no attempt will be made to save the patient's life—e.g., via CPR—once pulse and respirations cease. A person can use an advance directive form or tell the doctor that he doesn't want to be resuscitated. In this case, the doctor puts a DNR order on his medical chart.

Remember:

IF THE PATIENT HAS A LIVING WILL, DPA FOR HEALTH CARE, OR DNR, IT IS IMPORTANT THAT YOU PROVIDE HIS DOCTOR, OTHER FAMILY MEMBERS, THE HOSPITAL, AND EMERGENCY PERSONNEL (LOCAL AMBULANCE SERVICE) A COPY OF THE SIGNED DOCUMENTS/ORDERS.

Financial Issues

Inadequate finances may be a concern for the patient and his family. Lack of knowledge about the resources available may keep the patient from benefiting from the financial assistance he deserves. It is wise to investigate any options that may offer help.

Some Areas of Financial Assistance

SSI (Supplemental Security Income) is a program that provides a monthly income for people who are unable to meet their basic needs with the income they have. Medicaid and Food Stamps often supplement this income. The patient must be 65 years old or older, or be blind or disabled. To apply for SSI, contact the Social Security Administration, the local Area Agency on Aging or the local Department of Social Services.

General Assistance is a program that provides money or vouchers for rent, utilities, food, clothing, and medical care for people with very limited income. For more information, contact a legal services office or your local township office.

Food Stamp Program provides food stamps (coupons) that can be exchanged for food. Eligibility is based on need. For more information, contact the Department of Public Aid in the state in which the patient resides.

Medicaid* is a public aid program sponsored by the federal and state government that pays all or part of medical expenses. Eligibility requires that a person is 65 years old or older, or is blind or disabled, and have limited income. The Medicaid program covers many of the medical costs not covered by Medicare, such as prescription medications, and in some cases, long-term home health and in-home personal care. Each state sets its own income and asset eligibility requirements for Medicaid benefits.

Medicare is a federal health insurance program administered by the Social Security Administration for people who are 65 years old or older and some disabled people under age 65.

*Visit the Centers for Medicare/Medicaid Services web site at www.cms.gov for additional information about Medicaid.

Medicare pays for a portion of hospital and medical costs. At age 65, people are automatically enrolled if they receive Social Security or Railroad Retirement benefits. To inquire about the various services covered by Medicare, contact your local Social Security Office. Contact the patient's doctor, hospital, home health agency, or clinic to determine if they participate in the Medicare Program. Also ask if the patient's health care provider takes Medicare Assignment, which means they will accept the amount that Medicare approves to pay.

A **Medigap** policy is a health insurance policy sold by private insurance companies to fill the "gaps" in the Original Medicare Plan. Medigap policies help pay some of the health care costs that the Original Medicare Plan doesn't cover. If the patient is in the Original Medicare Plan and has a Medigap policy, then Medicare will pay its share and the Medigap policy will pay its share of health care costs.

Eligible U.S. military veterans can receive help to pay for health care provided at veteran's administration hospitals, adult day care services, in home assistance, and prescription medicines. Co-payments may be required and health insurance providers may be billed. For information, literature, eligibility standards, and to locate VA facilities in your area, call 1-800-872-1000 or call the Department of Veterans Affairs.

Other Programs

Tax deductions and credit are extended to "qualified individuals" who provide direct care for adults age 65 and older. Some items that may be tax deductible include transportation to medical appointments, privately hired in-home health aides, and changes to a residence or car for medical reasons. Adult day care expenses may be considered a medical deduction if the taxpayer itemizes using the appropriate IRS form. Contact the U.S. Internal

Revenue Service office listed in the local telephone directory for information or speak with a qualified accountant.

Meals and In-Home Services can help by providing home-delivered meals (Meals on Wheels) and home care services to those with limited income and resources. Contact the local Area Agency on Aging for more information about services available in your area.

Housing Assistance. The U.S. Department of Housing and Urban Development (HUD) offers rental assistance to eligible low-income residents of public or private housing units constructed and operated with HUD funds. Contact the county or city housing authority listed in the local telephone book. Information on Community Development Block Grants and loans for repairs and renovations are available to qualified urban home owners through local Community Development Offices. Check the telephone directory under "City Government" for a local community development office listing. There are also a number of U.S. Department of Agriculture Rural Housing Service programs for people living in rural areas. These range from loans to purchase a home, home-improvement and subsidy programs.

- Hospital Indemnity Policies pay a fixed amount of money for each day a person is hospitalized.
- Major Medical Policies cover the majority of the costs of medical treatment up to a certain amount.
- Health Maintenance Organizations (HMO) offer many services from preventive care to hospitalization.

Remember:

THE PATIENT CANNOT BE DENIED A MEDIGAP POLICY WITHIN THE FIRST 6 MONTHS OF MEDICARE ELIGIBILITY, REGARDLESS OF PAST OR PRESENT HEALTH STATUS.

Burial Trust Funds

A Burial Trust Fund can be established by depositing a predetermined amount of money into a fund available through most funeral homes. Funeral arrangements can also be made at the time a burial trust fund is opened. A prepaid, prearranged funeral takes the burden of making and paying for funeral arrangements from the family or guardian, at a time when they are feeling great loss. It is possible to set aside this money and not have it counted as an asset when applying for Medicaid.

☞ Remember:

ELDERCARE LOCATOR CAN PROVIDE YOU WITH ADDITIONAL INFORMATION ON MOST OF THE PROGRAMS AND ISSUES DISCUSSED IN THIS CHAPTER. SEE CHAPTER 14 FOR RESOURCE PHONE NUMBERS AND WEB SITES.

Summary

In summary, preparing an advance directive can give the patient a feeling of reassurance knowing that his wishes regarding medical care will be respected. There are three basic types of advance directive: the living will, durable power of attorney for healthcare (DOA) and do not resuscitate orders (DNR). As Medicare pays only a portion of medical costs, it may be wise to consider a health plan that will cover the expenses that Medicare does not.

in**sight**

Planning ahead can bring peace of mind.

Chapter 14

Resources

General Support Groups

Eldercare Locator

1-800-677-1116
Call between 9 am and 8 pm EST on weekdays. (Voice and TTY) See also the web site: www.eldercare.gov.

The Eldercare Locator is a free, national information and referral service of the Administration on Aging, U.S. Department of Health and Human Services, that directs callers to the appropriate state or local information sources for a variety of services. These services include legal assistance, housing options, adult day care, senior center programs, nursing home ombudsman, social and recreational activities, transportation, home-delivered meals, housekeeping, personal care, and home health care. When you call, you will be asked the senior citizen's zip code, city, residing county, and a brief description of the kind of help that is needed.

American Association of Retired Persons

601 E Street NW
Washington, D.C. 20049
1-800-687-2277 weekdays, 7:00 a.m. to midnight ET
www.aarp.org

American Health Assistance Foundation

A nonprofit charitable organization with over 30 years dedicated to funding research on Alzheimer's disease, glaucoma, macular degeneration, heart disease, and stroke.

22512 Gateway Center Dr
Clarksburg, MD 20871
www.ahaf.org

Children of Aging Parents

Children of Aging Parents is a nonprofit, charitable organization whose mission is to assist the nation's nearly 54 million caregivers of the elderly or chronically ill with reliable information, referrals and support, and to heighten public awareness that the health of the family caregivers is essential to ensure quality care of the nation's growing elderly population.

PO Box 167
Richboro, PA 18954
www.caps4caregivers.org

Hospice Foundation of America

Hospice Foundation of America provides leadership in the development and application of hospice and its philosophy of care with the goal of enhancing the American health care system and the role of hospice within it.

1-800-854-3402, Mon.-Fri., 9-5 EST
www.hospicefoundation.org

National Family Caregivers Association

The National Family Caregivers Association (NFCA) supports, empowers, educates, and speaks up for the more than 50 million Americans who care for a chronically ill, aged, or disabled loved one. NFCA reaches across the boundaries of different diagnoses, different relationships and different life stages to address the common needs and concerns of all family caregivers.

10400 Connecticut Avenue, Ste 500
Kensington, MD 20895-3944
1-800-896-3650
www.thefamilycaregiver.org

National Fraud Information Center

1-800-876-7060
Mon.-Fri., 9-5 EST
www.fraud.org

National Hospice and Palliative Care Organization

The National Hospice and Palliative Care Organization (NHPCO) is the largest nonprofit membership organization representing hospice and palliative care programs and professionals in the United States. The organization is committed to improving end of life care and expanding access to hospice care with the goal of profoundly enhancing quality of life for people dying in America and their loved ones.

1700 Diagonal Rd, Ste 625
Alexandria, VA 22314
1-703-837-1500
www.nhpco.org

Social Security Administration Online

The SSA pays retirement, disability and survivor's benefits to workers and their families and administers the Supplemental Security Income program. It also issues Social Security numbers.

Office of Public Inquiries
Windsor Park Building
6401 Security Blvd
Baltimore, MD 21235
1-800-772-1213 Mon.-Fri., 7-7 EST
www.ssa.gov

Department of Veterans Affairs

The VA's goal is to provide excellence in patient care, veterans' benefits and customer satisfaction. The department has been reformed internally and strives for high quality, prompt and seamless service to veterans. The department's employees continue to offer their dedication and commitment to help veterans get the services they have earned.

1-800-827-1000 (VA Benefits)
1-877-222-8387 (Health Care Benefits)
www.va.gov

Organizations for Specific Conditions

HIV/AIDS Treatment Information Service

AIDSinfo is a U.S. Department of Health and Human Services (DHHS) project that offers the latest federally approved information on HIV/AIDS clinical research, treatment and prevention, and medical practice guidelines for people living with HIV/AIDS, their families and friends, health care providers, scientists, and researchers.

Clinical Trials: AIDSinfo offers information on federally and privately funded clinical trials for AIDS patients and others infected with HIV. AIDS clinical trials evaluate experimental drugs and other therapies for adults and children at all stages of HIV infection - from patients who are HIV positive with no symptoms to those with various symptoms of AIDS.

Medical Guidelines: AIDSinfo serves as the main dissemination point for federally approved HIV treatment and prevention guidelines. AIDSinfo provides information about the current treatment regimens for HIV infection and AIDS-related illnesses, including the prevention of HIV transmission from occupational exposure and mother-to-child transmission during pregnancy.

AIDSinfo
PO Box 6303
Rockville, MD 20849-6303
Mon.-Fri., noon to 5 EST
www.aidsinfo.nih.gov

Alzheimer's Association

The Alzheimer's Association, the world leader in Alzheimer research and support, is the first and largest voluntary health organization dedicated to finding prevention methods, treatments and an eventual cure for Alzheimer's.

Alzheimer's Association National Office
225 N. Michigan Ave., Fl. 17
Chicago, Ill. 60601-7633
1-800-272-3900 24/7
www.alz.org

Alzheimer's Disease Education and Referral Center (ADEAR)

The U.S. Congress created the Alzheimer's Disease Education and Referral (ADEAR) Center in 1990 to "compile, archive, and disseminate information concerning Alzheimer's disease" for health professionals, people with AD and their families, and the public. The ADEAR Center is operated as a service of the National Institute on Aging (NIA), one of the Federal Government's National Institutes of Health and part of the U.S. Department of Health and Human Services. The NIA conducts and supports research about health issues for older people, and is the primary Federal agency for Alzheimer's disease research.

PO Box 8250
Silver Spring, MD 20907-8250
1-800-438-4380 Mon.-Fri., 8:30-5:00 EST
www.nia.nih.gov

Arthritis Foundation

The Arthritis Foundation is the only national not-for-profit organization that supports the more than 100 types of arthritis and related conditions with advocacy, programs, services and research.

PO Box 7669
Atlanta, GA 30357-0669
1-800-568-4045
www.arthritis.org

American Cancer Society

The American Cancer Society (ACS) is a nationwide, community-based voluntary health organization. Headquartered in Atlanta, Georgia, the ACS has state divisions and more than 3,400 local offices. Learn more about ACS, what it does, and its plans for the future by exploring the web site.

1-800-227-2345
www.cancer.org

American Diabetes Association

The American Diabetes Association is the nation's leading nonprofit health organization providing diabetes research, information and advocacy. Founded in 1940, the American Diabetes Association conducts programs in all 50 states and the District of Columbia, reaching hundreds of communities. The mission of the Association is to prevent and cure diabetes and to improve the lives of all people affected by diabetes.

To fulfill this mission, the American Diabetes Association funds research, publishes scientific findings, provides information and other services to people with diabetes, their families, health professionals and the public. The Association is also actively involved in advocating for scientific research and for the rights of people with diabetes.

www.diabetes.org

American Foundation for the Blind

The American Foundation for the Blind (AFB) is a national nonprofit that expands possibilities for people with vision loss. AFB's priorities include broadening access to technology; elevating the quality of information and tools for the professionals who serve people with vision loss; and promoting independent and healthy living for people with vision loss by providing them and their families with relevant and timely resources. AFB's work in these areas is supported by the strong presence the organization maintains in Washington, DC, ensuring the rights and interests of people with vision loss are represented in our nation's public policies.

11 Penn Plaza, Ste 300
New York, NY 10001
1-800-232-5463
www.afb.org

American Heart Association

The American Heart Association is a national voluntary health agency whose mission is to reduce disability and death from cardiovascular diseases and stroke.

7272 Greenville Ave
Dallas, TX 75231
www.americanheart.org

American Parkinson Disease Association

The American Parkinson Disease Association, Inc. was founded in 1961 to "ease the burden and find a cure" for Parkinson's disease. Headquartered in New York, the organization focuses its energies on research, patient support, education and raising public awareness of the disease.

135 Parkinson Ave
Staten Island, NY 10305
1-800-223-2732
www.apdaparkinson.org

American Speech-Language-Hearing Association (ASHA)

The mission of the American Speech-Language-Hearing Association is to promote the interests of and provide the highest quality services for professionals in audiology, speech-language pathology, and speech and hearing science, and to advocate for people with communication disabilities.

10801 Rockville Pike
Rockville, MD 20852
1-800-498-2071
www.asha.org

Cystic Fibrosis Foundation

The mission of the Cystic Fibrosis Foundation—a donor-supported, nonprofit organization—is to assure the development of the means to cure and control cystic fibrosis (CF) and to improve the quality of life for those with the disease.

6931 Arlington Rd
Bethesda, MD 20814
1-800-344-4823
www.cff.org

Epilepsy Foundation of America

The Epilepsy Foundation is the national voluntary agency solely dedicated to the welfare of the 2.7 million people with epilepsy in the U.S. and their families. The organization works to ensure that people with seizures are able to participate in all life experiences; and to prevent, control and cure epilepsy through research, education, advocacy and services. In addition to programs conducted at the national level, epilepsy clients throughout the United States are served by affiliated Epilepsy Foundation offices in nearly 100 communities.

www.epilepsyfoundation.org

Health Resources and Services Administration

The Health Resources and Services Administration (HRSA), an agency of the U.S. Department of Health and Human Services, is the primary Federal agency for improving access to health care services for people who are uninsured, isolated or medically vulnerable. Comprising five bureaus and 12 offices, HRSA provides leadership and financial support to health care providers in every state and U.S. territory.

5600 Fishers Lane
Rockville, MD 20857
1-800-638-0742
www.hrsa.gov

Leukemia Society of America

600 Third Ave., 4th Floor
New York, NY 10016
1-800-955-4572
www.leukemia.org

National Association for Continence (NAFC)

NAFC is the world's largest and most prolific consumer advocacy organization dedicated to public education and awareness about the causes, prevention, diagnosis, treatments, and management alternatives for incontinence.

PO Box 1019
Charleston, SC 29402-1019
1-800-252-3337
www.nafc.org

National Cancer Institute

The National Cancer Institute (NCI) is a component of the National Institutes of Health (NIH), one of eight agencies that compose the Public Health Service (PHS) in the Department of Health and Human Services (DHHS). The NCI, established under the National Cancer Act of 1937, is the Federal Government's principal agency for cancer research and training. The National Cancer Institute coordinates the National Cancer Program, which conducts and supports research, training, health information dissemination, and other programs with respect to the cause, diagnosis, prevention, and treatment of cancer, rehabilitation from cancer, and the continuing care of cancer patients and the families of cancer patients.

1-800-422-6237
www.cancer.gov

National Health Information Center

1-800-336-4797

National Institute of Mental Health(NIMH)

The NIMH mission is to reduce the burden of mental illness and behavioral disorders through research on mind, brain, and behavior. This public health mandate demands that we harness powerful scientific tools to achieve better understanding, treatment, and eventually, prevention of these disabling conditions that affect millions of Americans.

Public Information and Communications Branch
6001 Executive Blvd, Room 8184, MSC 9663
Bethesda, MD 20892-9663
www.nimh.nih.gov

National Institute of Neurological Disorders and Stroke (NINDS)

The mission of the NINDS is to reduce the burden of neurological disease—a burden borne by every age group, every segment of society, and people all over the world. To accomplish this goal the NINDS supports and conducts research, both basic and clinical, on the normal and diseased nervous system, fosters the training of investigators in the basic and clinical neurosciences, and seeks better understanding, diagnosis, treatment, and prevention of neurological disorders.

BRAIN
P.O. Box 5801
Bethesda, MD 20824
www.ninds.nih.gov

National Multiple Sclerosis Society

The Society and its network of chapters nationwide promote research, educate, advocate on critical issues, and organize a wide range of programs—including support for the newly diagnosed and those living with MS over time.

733 Third Ave
New York, NY 10017
1-800-344-4867
www.nmss.org

United Cerebral Palsy

United Cerebral Palsy (UCP) is the leading source of information on cerebral palsy and is a pivotal advocate for the rights of persons with any disability. As one of the largest health charities in America, the UCP mission is to advance the independence, productivity and full citizenship of people with disabilities through an affiliate network.

1660 L St, NW, Ste 700
Washington, DC 20036
www.ucp.org

United Ostomy Associations of America, Inc.

UOAA is a national network for bowel and urinary diversion support groups in the United States. Its goal is to provide a nonprofit association that will serve to unify and strengthen its member support groups, which are organized for the benefit of people who have, or will have intestinal or urinary diversions and their caregivers.

1-800-826-0826
www.uoaa.org

Y-ME Breast Cancer Support Program

Y-ME National Breast Cancer Organization (Y-ME) is a Chicago-based national nonprofit organization with the mission to ensure, through information, empowerment and peer support, that no one faces breast cancer alone. Y-ME does not raise money for research.

1-800-221-2141 (24 hour hotline)
www.y-me.org

Additional Services

To locate additional services in your community, check your yellow page directory and contact: the American Red Cross, Visiting Nurses Association, YMCA, United Way, home care agencies, churches or synagogues, local hospitals, public health departments, nursing homes, civic, social, or volunteer organizations, housing departments, or county extension office.

Also check your telephone directory for a section on Community Services by category.

Parish nursing is a health ministry that functions as a resource and referral service promoting health care while incorporating the emotional, intellectual, social, physical, and spiritual well-being of the individuals they serve. By showing the love of God, health nursing and ministries work to promote holistic health for members of their congregations. Call your local place of worship to determine if this service is available in your area.

Adult day care programs consist of various structured services and activities designed to maximize independence for the patient and provide temporary relief for the caregiver.

Adult day care programs offer an opportunity for the older or disabled adult to maintain a sense of community and self-worth. Participants include persons who could benefit from socialization while receiving assistance with activities of daily living. Referrals for adult day care can be made by the patient, family, friends, caregiver, clergy, social worker or other health care professional. Also, you can check the yellow pages of the phone book under "day care" for resources in your area.

You can obtain a wealth of useful information for both yourself and the person you are caring for from your local **public library**. The reference librarian can help you access information from books or the Internet on government publications and health-related organizations that may not be included in this chapter.

M

N

O

P

R

S

T

U

V

W

Y